A PLUME BOOK

FAT FAMILY / FIT FAMILY

The MORELLIS are a family that struggled with obesity—and conquered it. In January 2009, Ron Morelli and his eighteen-year-old son, Mike, were cast as contestants on season seven of *The Biggest Loser*, making it to the final four and losing four hundred pounds combined. At home, Becky (who has previously lost 125 pounds) and her youngest son, Max, watched with America as her family shrank. Inspired by his father's and brother's success, Max went on to lose almost 150 pounds. Now, the formerly fat family has become a fit family, inspiring millions along the way. The Morellis live in South Lyon, Michigan, and continue to educate others about nutrition, fitness, and weight loss.

FAT FAMILY / FIT FAMILY

HOW WE BEAT OBESITY AND YOU CAN TOO

Ron, Becky, Mike, and Max Morelli

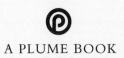

A PLUME BOOK

PLUME
Published by the Penguin Group
Penguin Group (USA) Inc., 375 Hudson Street, New York, New York 10014, U.S.A. • Penguin
Group (Canada), 90 Eglinton Avenue East, Suite 700, Toronto, Ontario, Canada M4P 2Y3
(a division of Pearson Penguin Canada Inc.) • Penguin Books Ltd., 80 Strand, London WC2R 0RL,
England • Penguin Ireland, 25 St. Stephen's Green, Dublin 2, Ireland (a division of Penguin Books
Ltd.) • Penguin Group (Australia), 250 Camberwell Road, Camberwell, Victoria 3124, Australia
(a division of Pearson Australia Group Pty. Ltd.) • Penguin Books India Pvt. Ltd., 11 Community
Centre, Panchsheel Park, New Delhi – 110 017, India • Penguin Group (NZ), 67 Apollo Drive,
Rosedale, North Shore 0632, New Zealand (a division of Pearson New Zealand Ltd.) • Penguin
Books (South Africa) (Pty.) Ltd., 24 Sturdee Avenue, Rosebank, Johannesburg 2196, South Africa

Penguin Books Ltd., Registered Offices: 80 Strand, London WC2R 0RL, England

First published by Plume, a member of Penguin Group (USA) Inc.

First Printing, April 2011
10 9 8 7 6 5 4 3 2 1

Ⓟ REGISTERED TRADEMARK—MARCA REGISTRADA

LIBRARY OF CONGRESS CATALOGING-IN-PUBLICATION DATA

Morelli, Ron.
    Fat family/fit family : how we beat obesity and you can too / Ron Morelli . . . [et.al.].
        p. cm.
    ISBN 978-0-452-29693-0 (pbk. : alk. paper)   1. Obesity—Prevention.   2. Weight loss.
3. Nutrition. 4.   Physical fitness.   I. Title.
    RA645.O23M68 2011
    613.2'5—dc22

                                                                              2010051998

Printed in the United States of America
Set in Bembo
Designed by Eve L. Kirch

PUBLISHER'S NOTE
The Biggest Loser is not associated with this book or any of the views or information contained in
this book.

Every effort has been made to ensure that the information contained in this book is complete and
accurate. However, neither the publisher nor the author is engaged in rendering professional advice
or services to the individual reader. The ideas, procedures, and suggestions contained in this book
are not intended as a substitute for consulting with your physician. All matters regarding your
health require medical supervision. Neither the author nor the publisher shall be liable or respon-
sible for any loss or damage allegedly arising from any information or suggestion in this book.

Penguin is committed to publishing works of quality and integrity.
In that spirit, we are proud to offer this book to our readers;
however, the story, the experiences, and the words
are the authors' alone.

This book is dedicated to everyone who has struggled—or is still struggling—to beat obesity.

Never give up! You can change your life!

Contents

Acknowledgments

Ron: I must thank my mother for never giving up on me, supporting me on so many screwball diets, taking me to so many diet doctors, always trying to help, and always believing that I would someday live a healthier life.

I have tremendous gratitude for my trainer on *The Biggest Loser*, Bob Harper, who made me realize that I'm not too old and that I can still do whatever I set my mind to. He pushed me further than I thought I could be pushed, through the pain and into an amazing new life.

A huge thank-you goes to the producers of *The Biggest Loser* for blessing our family with better health and happiness than we could ever imagine.

I can't even express how much I love and appreciate my wife and kids, who supported me through bypass surgery, the show, and everything else in our lives. Thank you for loving me whether I was 500 pounds or 250 pounds.

I am forever grateful to the St. John Providence Health System, South Lyon Area Recreation Authority, South Lyon Community Schools, and Anytime Fitness for opening your doors for the Morelli Health and Fitness Camp. Thank you to all the families who entrusted Michael and me to help your children lose weight, and thanks to the kids: we appreciate that you worked so hard to feel better!

Becky: I want to first thank my family for achieving our dream of becoming fit.

And I must say thank you to the producers of *The Biggest Loser*, who found Mike's and Ron's stories compelling and engaging. They took a chance on our family and selected Mike and Ron as the lucky ones. As a result, we are forever changed, with many years of healthier, happier living to enjoy together.

My heartfelt thanks to my parents for always loving me, never judging me, and for wanting the best for me.

To Ron, Michael, and Max: I appreciate you even more for never giving up and for sticking to your programs until you saw the results you wished for.

Mike: I have an incredible new life, and I have to first thank my dad for agreeing to go to *The Biggest Loser* audition with me. Thank you, beyond words, to the producers who gave us the chance to re-create ourselves. Bob Harper and Jillian Michaels—you are both amazing, and I will always appreciate you immensely.

My deepest thanks goes to Jimi Varner—personal trainer, mentor, and friend—who helped me build on what I learned at the ranch and apply it in my real life. His knowledge, encouragement, and support continue to be a driving force behind my physical fitness and strength of character, for which I am forever grateful.

Mom, thank you for always believing that someday I would reveal the healthy, happy young man that was hiding inside me for so many years.

Max, you were my eating buddy; now you're my living buddy, because we're having a blast!

Max: I have to thank my family first for believing that even though I was the last one to lose weight, I would still someday succeed.

I'm thankful that *The Biggest Loser* helped my dad and brother, because their success inspired mine.

And of course, thank you so, so much to the owners of the Biggest Loser Resort at Fitness Ridge, where I literally left behind nearly 150 pounds of my old life as I stepped into my new one.

And thank you to all my friends, who've been there for me whether I was obese or not.

From all of us: Thank you, Elizabeth Atkins, for composing our stories into this book, something we could never have done ourselves.

Another thanks goes to publicist Kristin Schenden for always giving great guidance about how to share our story.

A huge thank-you goes out to our community of South Lyon, Michigan, for the overwhelmingly positive support that friends and strangers alike have shown for us over the years and since the show. You make us proud to live in South Lyon.

A very special thank-you goes to literary agent Barbara Lowenstein and editors Cherise Fisher and Kate Napolitano for believing in our story and enabling us to share it with the world.

Introduction

food·a·hol·ic—*noun:* a person having an excessive, often uncontrollable craving for food.

—Dictionary.com

What do you get when two foodaholics get married?

A fat family.

A dad whose weight spiked over five hundred pounds.

Two teenagers, both nearly four hundred pounds.

And a mother, who, after beating her own obesity, then tried desperately for years to stop her husband and sons from eating themselves to death.

That was us: Ron, Becky, Michael, and Max.

The Morelli family.

Like millions of American parents and kids right now, we lived to eat—as much, and as often, as we could. Food was love. Food was happiness and fun family time. Food was comfort.

Food was our addiction.

We lived for those lost-in-the-moment highs as burgers and ice cream and cookies and pizza and fried foods had a party with our taste buds and filled our bellies well beyond satisfaction.

Whether our appetites were stoked by stress, bad habits, cravings, or some deep emotional yearning, food was the ultimate
feel-good remedy. All day, every day, it was our legal, socially
celebrated drug of choice.

And we hated it.

We hated the misery, the fat, the discomfort, the health problems, the self-disgust, and the guilt. Worst of all, we hated the
hopeless feeling that we could never control our eating enough
to lose weight and stay thin. We hated the overwhelming idea
that it would take forever and a day to diet and exercise away
hundreds of pounds. We prayed for an extreme solution that
would change our lives forever.

Little did we know, our prayers would be answered—in front
of millions of TV viewers around the world.

"*The Biggest Loser* is having auditions here," eighteen-year-old
Michael announced in our kitchen one evening in June 2008. "I
heard it on the radio on the way to work."

"I heard that commercial too," said Ron, who'd watched
every episode of the hit NBC prime-time show since its premiere.

"Me too," added Max, who had recently finished his sophomore year of high school. "The show's looking for teams."

"I also heard it," said Becky, while preparing her usual vegetables and Egg Beaters. Since losing 125 pounds after gastric
bypass surgery twelve years before, she'd usually eaten the same
dinner every day before taking a walk around the neighborhood.

The kitchen fell silent. You could almost see a lightbulb going
off in our heads as we stood around the kitchen island—the same
counter where we'd eaten countless meals and snacks that we
were literally still wearing as fat.

Could *The Biggest Loser* finally help the Morelli men lose
weight and keep it off? "Let's try out, Dad," said Michael.

Mike
Desperate for Change

I was only eighteen, but I weighed almost 400 pounds. I'd gained 150 pounds in high school alone. I had just graduated from Detroit Catholic Central High School with a 3.9 GPA and was headed to Michigan State University in the fall. Despite good grades and good friends, I was worried. How could I enjoy college when I loathed everything about my body? Being obese had squashed my self-esteem; I dreaded going to college, where I was bound to make a horrible first impression in my premed classes, in the dorm, and at parties.

I was so grossly overweight that I needed an extreme solution. Standing in the kitchen in my size 56 jeans, I reflected on my eating habits: I worked at McDonald's, where I'd not only eaten breakfast, lunch, and dinner but snacked on chicken nuggets like they were popcorn. I had easily consumed five thousand calories, without even blinking an eye, and the day wasn't over.

Another summer was here: another summer during which I wouldn't dare bare my sixty-five-inch waist at a pool or beach; another summer with sweat forming in the folds of fat on my back.

Being fat and eating huge amounts of food had been my identity for as long as I could remember. And it wasn't always bad. Some of my happiest memories are of Christmas at my grandma's house, where everybody was having a great time and eating like there was no tomorrow. We feasted on homemade Italian food from a huge buffet: lasagna, spaghetti and meatballs, sausage, pizza, breadsticks, roast beef, and cannoli. The basement was set up like a banquet hall, with Frank Sinatra playing as dozens of relatives feasted in celebration of life and family. You could feel the love just exploding in the house, and food was an expression of that love.

Dad and all my uncles were really big men who devoured enormous portions. Max and I looked up to them as strong and masculine; we wanted to be just like Dad. So we always refilled our plates at least three times.

For both of us, it was cool to be "the big kid" until middle school, when we both became "the fat kid." Being an obese teenager was miserable.

I prayed that *The Biggest Loser* would be my escape. I'd seen the trainers work contestants so hard that they puked and cried. If that's what it would take to transform me from a fat foodaholic into a normal-weight person, then I was ready.

Max
Hoping to Audition Too

As we stood around the kitchen, I could feel everyone's excitement. For me, going on a TV show sounded like it would be a blast. And shrinking my body down to a size where I could play sports and wear cool clothes and move around as easily as my thin friends? Well, that sounded amazing. But it also sounded like an impossible dream that I'd never been able to achieve. I just couldn't see myself giving up the lifestyle I'd known for as long as I could remember.

I loved food—lots and lots of it, all day long and into the night. I didn't like limits or boundaries.

Feasting on great food was fun for us Morellis. We were always going out to eat, or Dad was bringing home a pizza from work, or we were taking a vacation with endless snacks and meals. Eating with my family meant no judgment, just pure enjoyment. And we were so caught up in that enjoyment that it was easy to ignore the fact that our fun was also causing our misery.

While hanging out with friends in high school, food was

always the focus of our fun. We'd go out for Mexican, or chicken wings, and then sit around watching TV or playing video games. I'd been a Little League baseball star back in elementary school, but weighing two hundred pounds in fifth grade meant my sports days were numbered. Like Michael, I played freshman football in high school, but after that I was just too fat to play.

Being obese was the only hugely negative thing about my life. I had great friends, loving parents, and a nice house; went to private school and on family vacations; had a car that Michael and I shared, and all the latest video games. At school I was known for being the life of the party because I did things like paint myself blue and cheer the loudest of anybody at basketball and football games. But nobody saw the times at home when I would cry to my mom because I was so fat.

The fatter I got, the more I felt like all the normal, fun stuff teenagers are supposed to do was passing me by. Especially with girls. They loved me—as a friend. Not as a boyfriend. That depressed me, so I'd eat more and get bigger. I needed a huge change. Unfortunately, as we stood around the kitchen contemplating what seemed like a magic solution, I realized it wasn't for me. According to the radio commercial I'd heard, I was too young to audition. But if Dad and Michael got on *The Biggest Loser*, I wondered, could that help me too?

RON
I Had to Save My Sons

"Let's give it a try," I said that fateful evening in our kitchen. "We'll audition. What's the worst thing that can happen? We waste a day. But at least we'll have tried."

Doing the physically grueling challenges that were part of the show seemed impossible for a sick, broken-down guy like me. But at that point, I would do anything to spare Michael and Max from my miserable fate.

Five decades of stuffing my body with food was killing me. At fifty-four I was shooting myself up with insulin and taking four-teen pills a day for diabetes, high blood pressure, hypertension, and high cholesterol. I had to sleep with a mask connected to a machine because the fat squeezing my throat and chest made me stop breathing at night. And excruciating pain continually shot through my knees.

I'd tried every weight-loss gimmick out there, from shakes and pills to having my jaw wired shut for six months. Another time, I sold my house, my car, and my business to pay for a long stay at a residential weight-loss center. I'd dropped more than a hundred pounds every time I'd started on one of those plans—*five times already!*—but I'd always gained it back, and then some.

Even gastric bypass surgery hadn't kept me thin! It'd been thirteen years since surgeons had reduced my stomach to the size of an egg.

But a foodaholic always pushes the limits. After the operation I was supposed to eat only low-fat, pureed foods while my stom-ach adapted. I couldn't stick to that: once I actually pureed a Big Mac in the food processor! And by sampling a french fry here or a cookie there, I forced my tiny stomach to tolerate fatty foods and stretched the opening to my small intestine. It wasn't long before I was back to my favorite chili-drenched hot dogs, pizza, and my mother's home-cooked Italian food.

So there I was, huge and pretty hopeless, and my son wanted me to go on national TV and expose it all. Male contestants on *The Biggest Loser* wore nothing but shorts as they did the most humiliating thing for a heavy person: to get weighed, and for the entire world to watch!

But somehow I had to save myself and my sons. Still, *The Biggest Loser* felt like a fantasy, like when the lottery is up to $300 million and you think, "Oh, I should buy a ticket," but you don't. The odds seemed one in a million that we'd get picked.

BECKY
I Didn't Think It Would Happen

Ron could hardly get around the house. How would he be able to exercise in *The Biggest Loser* gym and do those crazy challenges? I would watch him struggling and think, "No wonder you can't move—you're so fat."

I never said that. Ron's weight was like an elephant in the room that nobody talked about. However, it had been our favorite subject when we'd met, twenty-one years before, at a residential weight-loss center. Happy and in love, we had vowed to never get big again. But when the boys were small, I'd blown up to 260 pounds (I'm five foot seven). So when Michael was in first grade and Max was in preschool, I also had gastric bypass surgery. Thankfully, I lost 125 pounds, and I'd kept it off for thirteen years.

But Ron had gone back to eating like it was an Olympic sport. And the boys had sided with him, eating thousands of extra calories every day, ballooning toward four hundred pounds each.

As we talked about *The Biggest Loser*, I didn't want us to get our hopes up, only to have them smashed by disappointment. But I was also thinking, "We have to do something before Michael and Max end up like Ron."

FIT FAMILY
If We Did the Impossible, So Can You

"Pack your bags for five months," the producer said, when he called in three months after Michael and Ron auditioned. "Because you're coming to California."

But once there, we still had to compete with ninety-eight other people for just twenty-two spots on the show. The anxiety ended when the show's host, Alison Sweeney, told us, "You're going to the ranch!"

Now, thanks to that extraordinary experience, we are a fit family.

But it isn't easy. They say, "Once an alcoholic, always an alcoholic," because one sip can set off that insatiable craving that drowns all self-control. Well, we could say, "Once a foodaholic, always a foodaholic." But the difference is that an alcoholic can stop drinking forever; foodaholics, however, must still eat, at least three times a day.

Sometimes we struggle to resist urges to indulge in old favorites like cookies, pizza, burgers, and fries. But we feel so much better now that we never want to go back to the unhealthy misery of being obese. As a result, we're winning the battle against our foodaholic past.

We've done what millions of American families dream of doing. That's why we're sharing our story, to show how we transformed from a fat family with a food addiction into a fit family committed to healthy eating, exercising, and living a life far better than we ever imagined.

You might think it's impossible, but you *can* beat obesity. If our family did it, so can yours.

—Ron, Becky, Mike, and Max Morelli

FAT FAMILY/ FIT FAMILY

CHAPTER **1** / **RON**

It Was Love at First Sight

If you had seen me back in 1987, when I was thirty-two, the words "tall, dark, and handsome" would probably not have come to mind. Sure, I was six feet tall. I had "dark" covered with my full beard and shoulder-length black hair. And some women even said I was handsome.

But I weighed nearly five hundred pounds.

And I was miserable.

I wasn't living. I was existing. All I did was work, eat, and sleep.

So I gave myself an ultimatum: either slay the foodaholic beast within or allow my self-destructive compulsion to continue squeezing the life out of me, literally and figuratively.

The choice was clear. I had to beat my lifetime battle with obesity once and for all. I wanted to feel excited about life. I wanted to fall in love and share my future with a wonderful woman who loved me for me.

And I knew just where I could make that happen.

With spring in full bloom, I checked myself into a weight-loss center in Durham, North Carolina. Durham is known as the diet capital of the world because so many weight-loss clinics are located there.

As I entered the building designed to look like an old southern home, I was a man on a mission. Passing through those white double doors into the cozy home-style lobby, I beamed with confidence—even euphoria—that yes, *this time* I would finally end my struggle with food and fat, and live a happy life as a thin guy.

I knew I could do it, because I'd done it once. Two years before, I'd lost more than a hundred pounds here at Structure House. The weight had fallen off so easily and quickly that I'd wowed the staff and inspired the clients. No one had been more thrilled than me, because after a lifetime of being obese, "thin Ron" was finally within reach.

But that dream had disappeared just as fast.

Spending eight hundred to one thousand dollars every week for five months had bankrupted me. So I returned home to suburban Detroit, still weighing well over 300 pounds. I stuffed down burgers, fries, cookies, pizzas, and home-cooked Italian food until I gained 150 pounds. Fast.

Now I was back at Structure House for the second time. With the beautiful tulips and magnolias, it was the perfect season to escape my gloom and finally shine as the happy, successful person I was supposed to become.

That was my first wish. My second wish was to meet a woman who would share that new life with me. Just hours after arriving, I walked into orientation in a gymnasium with about a hundred overweight and obese people, and caught sight of a pretty brunette in jeans and a red blouse. Something about her was radiant and comforting; I felt a connection on a visceral level. I knew my second wish would come true too.

"I'm going to marry that girl," I told a stranger beside me. I had never been surer of anything. It didn't matter that I was not the typical eligible bachelor. Structure House was different from the real world, where being fat often makes you a social outcast. When everyone around you is overweight or obese, "real world" standards of beauty don't apply. Instead you're judged by your personality.

At Structure House, making friends came naturally. Everyone around you shared a similar disposition. When I told a guy named Harry that I weighed 487 pounds, he shot back, jokingly, in his heavy New Jersey accent, "What's the matter with you? Couldn't you just gain 13 more and join the nickel club?"

Harry was almost as big as me, but older, and we became instant buddies. That first night I joined him and a half-dozen people, including a woman named Pepper, in the southern-style dining room. I was delighted when the mesmerizing brunette approached our table where her friends had joined us.

After Pepper introduced us, Becky said, "We're playing water volleyball tonight. Do you want to play?"

I felt like Cupid had just shot me up with a bunch of arrows. I was love-struck. Becky was twenty-three and from Atlanta, Georgia. She had graduated from Emory University with a degree in marketing. At 210 pounds, she was one of the thinner people there. And she was perfect. I learned that she'd been at orientation to help greet newcomers; she had already been there for a week.

"My group is going home," Becky said playfully, "so I need to start being nice to other people so I can have some friends." New groups of ten or fifteen people arrived every seven days, while others left. You could stay as long as you wanted, if you kept paying the eight hundred to a thousand dollars every week for meals, lectures, group and individual therapy, nutrition classes, exercise activities, and lodging in apartments.

I laughed, and when I looked into Becky's blue eyes I saw a twinkle that left no doubt: Cupid's arrow had struck her too.

That night we all played water volleyball in the pool. It might sound weird for a bunch of heavy people to get excited about putting on bathing suits—something many normal-weight people dread. But when everybody's big, nobody really cares. Plus the water is up to your chest, and at Structure House, everyone is confident that in a matter of weeks or months they will be much thinner. We had an absolute ball, even inviting a few well-known actors who were there to join our game.

After that night, Becky and I became inseparable.

We spent seventeen hours a day together. In the morning we left our respective apartments and walked in groups through the pretty, tree-lined streets of Durham. Then we went to breakfast in the dining room. That was usually an egg-white omelet with mushrooms, a slice of dry toast, and strawberry sorbet.

During the day, we talked with a psychologist, in groups and individually, about why we were so addicted to food. In nutrition seminars, we learned about balancing fat, carbohydrates, and protein. And we burned tons of calories in exercise classes. Afterward Becky and I would take romantic walks through the botanical gardens at nearby Duke University.

Falling in love with Becky was as close to a fairy tale as I'd ever get. In fact, our first date was to see the movie *Snow White*. I asked her out when we went with a dozen friends to see *The Rocky Horror Picture Show* at the local theater. We couldn't sit together, but later, I referred to the preview we'd seen for *Snow White*. "We should go see that."

"Okay," Becky said eagerly. Another time we saw *Harry and the Hendersons*, but we could've been watching paint dry, because it was thrilling to be together.

Nighttime was the best. I went to Becky's apartment on the Structure House campus (my apartment was off-campus), and we would talk for hours, about everything.

After years of feeling fat, lonely, and unacceptable, it was incredible to connect with a pretty girl who wanted to know everything about me. She liked me for me, and that was the best feeling in the world. Over the course of our three-month stay, I shared the most intimate details of my life with her.

I WAS ALWAYS BIG

Peanut butter.

Boy, did I love peanut butter as a kid. When I was about five years old, in the late 1950s, it seemed like that big glass jar of Velvet-brand peanut butter would call my name from the kitchen cabinet. Since Mom was so busy with a new baby and three toddlers, and Dad was at work, I would sneak into the small green kitchen at the front of our ranch-style home.

My heart would pound with anticipation as I lifted the jar from the shelf. Then, as I unscrewed the lid, I got even more excited at the sight of the smooth, untouched surface with a little dollop where a machine had filled the jar.

I was totally lost in the moment as I inhaled the salty-sweet scent. I'd plunge a spoon into the soft surface, scoop up a creamy glob, raise it to my mouth, and savor it as it melted on my tongue. Sweet, salty, creamy, rich. I was never happier than when I was eating peanut butter. Of course, I was always listening to make sure Ma wouldn't walk in and catch me sneaking food between meals.

Years later she would tell me that I had been a normal weight until I was four. But at age five I had started to pack on the pounds—and never stopped. It was no wonder, as I secretly binged on one of the most fattening foods you can eat. But as a kid I had no concept of calories or fat. I just had an overwhelming desire to eat as often and as much as I could.

As my taste buds had a flavor fest under globs of peanut butter, my eyes would drift to the yellow label on the jar. Below the letters that spelled out "Velvet" in a blue, green, and red accordion of jesterlike squares were three little guys' faces and the words "creamy peanut butter."

Even today, if you look at a jar of Velvet Peanut Butter, you'll see my three little binge buddies: One, beside the word "fresh," looks mischievous and mad. Below him, the middle boy, next to "pure," has a halo. And the third guy is licking his lips beside "delicious."

That image became forever imprinted in my mind because the little guys' expressions would ultimately mirror back my feelings about food—as a kid and even now that I'm well into my fifties. But at the time, my only thought was that it tasted good, and I wanted to enjoy that feeling for as long as possible.

FOOD WAS MY ESCAPE

My mother came home from the hospital with a new baby *seven times* before my tenth birthday. As devout Catholics, my mother and father, whose parents emigrated from Italy, believed in having as many children as God would provide. So when I was one year old, my sister was born. On my second birthday, another sister arrived. Then came five more babies. Eight kids in ten years.

Imagine all those babies, toddlers, and kids, with cribs, playpens, toys, strollers, and car seats, crammed into our 1,800-square-foot house in Lathrup Village, which at the time was a new suburb of Detroit, Michigan. We had one bathroom and three bedrooms; the girls shared a room, and the boys had a room with two double beds.

As the oldest kid, I was the babysitter, the diaper changer, the clean-up crew, and the mediator when my siblings bickered. If one of them did something and got yelled at, I got yelled at too, because it happened on my watch. It was rare when you could be by yourself and not worry about what someone else was doing.

I had no privacy. No alone time. Except when I was secretly eating. Food was the one thing that didn't cry, didn't need a diaper changed, wasn't yelling at you, wasn't taking your toys.

Food was my escape. Even if the pleasure lasted only a minute or two—when I'd sneak a piece of chicken from the refrigerator or a cookie from the cabinet—eating made me feel happy. Food was my best friend. It gave me comfort when I was by myself. As the tastes and textures delighted my senses, everything was okay. Not that the rest was bad. It just wasn't as good as eating.

I was always thinking about what I would eat next. I guess I was born into the right family, because for my grandmothers and my mother food was everything. They were never happier than when they were feeding you. For them, the kitchen was the heart of the home. They began preparing dinner in the morning, making everything from scratch. The house smelled heavenly all day long.

Peppers bubbled in olive oil on the stove, while garlic-and-herb-rubbed roast or chicken or Italian bread baked in the oven. Made-from-scratch tomato sauce simmered on the stovetop too. All this tantalized my taste buds from the moment I arrived home from school.

Dinner was at five thirty every day. Being late was a cardinal sin in the Morelli family. We each had our own spot around the table, and we ate family-style, after my father said grace and my mother covered the brown Formica table with huge platters. A typical dinner would include pasta with tomato sauce, vegetables, and meat—usually baked chicken, turkey, ham, or roast beef—and salad with my mother's homemade vinaigrette. She also made the best lasagna, spaghetti, meatballs, and cannoli you could ever imagine.

We kids even handpicked some of the ingredients. During the summer, my parents and grandparents would take us to these big farms in rural Michigan to pick tomatoes. Then the adults would make and can enough sauce for the year, and they'd roast a twelve-month supply of peppers to keep in the freezer. We also had a garden, where Ma would get fresh herbs, tomatoes, and cucumbers to serve during the warmer months.

Food was love, and Ma lavished it on us at every meal. She put all her efforts into making sure we had the most delicious foods in front of us. But you had to grab it fast, or you wouldn't eat—not with ten people around the table and twenty hands reaching for my mother's home-cooked magic! At the end of the meal, the food was gone. If she made a four-pound roast, we'd eat four pounds of roast. If she prepared a six-pound roast, we'd eat six pounds.

Sometimes she'd bake five chickens, and all the kids loved the wings. We'd each take one. While my brothers and sisters were bickering over who'd get the remaining two, I'd eat them. End of argument.

Our father was quiet as he ate at the head of the table, tired from getting up at 5:00 a.m. to work at a construction job that he hated but went to every day of his life. Muscular and swarthy, with a perpetual five o'clock shadow, he had eight kids by the time he was thirty-five.

After serving in the United States Army at the end of World War II, Dad abandoned his dream of going to college and becoming an architect. Instead he did what a good Italian son was supposed to do: work with his father in the family business, in this case a small excavating company. Dad was all about work and responsibility and providing for his family.

My father's whole life was work. He hated winter, but he worked in snow and frigid temperatures for four or five months of the year. If a rainstorm or blizzard struck, he couldn't work, which meant he didn't get paid. Even our summer vacations revolved around work: we'd rent a cottage in northern Michigan in places where he could take construction jobs.

His workday always ended with the same ritual. He'd come home, enter through the garage, and go to the basement. He'd remove his dusty work clothes that reeked of diesel fuel from the cranes and other heavy machinery he operated. He'd change into clean clothes, and then come upstairs for dinner. By the time he sat down with us, he must have been too tired and have had too many worrisome things on his mind to chitchat about what we'd done all day at school, where his hard work paid the tuition. It was our stay-at-home mother who would ask, "Ronald, how was school today?"

As you can imagine, it was pretty noisy in our house. I used to get horrible earaches. As a result, I had four or five operations, including a tonsillectomy and the insertion of a mastoid bone from a cadaver in my left ear. The earaches stopped, but they left me legally deaf in that ear. Of course I could still hear the noise that my brothers and sisters usually made together.

"You have buck teeth!" someone would taunt.

"You have frizzy hair!" someone would shoot back.

Even though I was the chubby one, I don't remember them making fun of my weight. And if kids at school poked fun at me, it was behind my back.

We had a comfortable life because our parents worked hard every day. If you had to describe my parents in a few words, it would be "dutiful" and "devoted," to family and church. Every Sunday my mother corralled the eight of us—babies, toddlers, and kids—into a pew at St. Bede Catholic Church. Dad was an usher, so he did not sit with us. During the service, I would look forward to the big Sunday dinner we would enjoy later. Then, like every night of the week, we older kids would clear the table, do the dishes, and sweep the floor.

"Ronald," my mother would say, "watch your brothers and sisters while I get the babies ready for bed."

I would do as I was told, looking forward to the opportunity to sneak back into the kitchen to grab a cookie.

FOOD BRINGS PLEASURE AND PAIN

When I was nine years old, I loved playing football. Since I was so big, the coaches put me on a team with twelve-year-old boys who'd been playing in our city's parks and recreation league for three or four years. The rule was that boys in that group could play only if we weighed a maximum of two hundred pounds in our gear.

At first it was cool to be so young and be the big kid on the team. I also loved that my dad took time away from work to come to the games. But as the other boys were growing stronger and faster, I was getting fatter and slower. I went from being the star on the team to being the last one picked, unless we were playing tug-of-war, in which case I was suddenly every team's top pick.

Each year the kids trying out for the team had to step on a scale to make sure they qualified for the weight class. Each year

I'd dread it. When I was ten years old, in fifth grade, I stepped on the scale and was shocked. I had exceeded the two-hundred-pound limit. The coaches told me I had to stop playing football because I was too heavy. It was one of the worst moments of my childhood. How ironic that, years later, I would revisit this trauma by stepping on a scale in front of millions of people on television! As a kid, though, I coped by burying myself in the very thing that caused the problem in the first place. Like the alcoholic who didn't get the job because he had booze on his breath, then leaves the interview and gets drunk, a foodaholic goes on an eating rampage when he's disappointed or sad. Rejected from the local football team, I ate to comfort myself. Peanut butter, cookies, pasta, you name it—I ate it. During those fleeting moments when I was eating, I felt good. But then I went right back to the misery, because the eating high only lasts a moment: after you finish gorging, you're still fat.

With eight kids in the house, we were constantly going through food, so no one seemed to notice if I sneaked a bite here or there. It wasn't unusual for us to have ten or twelve boxes of cereal in the cabinet at once. And it's not as if my brothers and sisters didn't snack too. But the difference between me and the other kids was that, no matter how much they ate, they never gained weight. They were all thin. "Geez," I wondered, "why aren't they putting on weight too?"

When I was ten, we moved into a much bigger house, three miles away in a brand new neighborhood in Southfield. Our 2,800-square-foot colonial had five bedrooms, a family room with a wet bar, a formal dining room, and a first-floor laundry with a sewing room. The exterior was red brick with white aluminum siding upstairs and black shutters, and there was a giant tree on the front lawn.

Southfield was mostly Jewish, but we lived in a small pocket of

Catholic families. When another Italian family moved in behind us, I developed my first crush, on Michelle, who was also ten.

"Someday, when you grow up, you'll get married to each other," our mothers would say playfully. I felt shy and never believed someone as pretty as Michelle would want a guy who weighed twice as much as most kids our age.

Some of my happiest times were going to "the yard" where my dad and my grandfather kept heavy equipment near a trailer-type office. I was awed when they dug a basement next to my grand-parents' house in Detroit. Dad was so strong; once he put one hand on a waist-high chain-link fence and leaped over it. In my eyes, he was Superman. As we kids watched him and Grandpa work, I thought, "Boy, is that ever great! I wanna be just like them."

But I wasn't: I was fat and getting fatter. My dad, however, treated me like all the other kids. He wasn't a warm and fuzzy guy, but he made sure we had wholesome family fun. In the win-ter, he'd take us to a local park where they had bonfires, skating rinks, doughnuts, and cider. Then we'd take rides down a hill on an eight-foot toboggan that he bought for us to ride together.

Despite all this activity, I kept gaining weight.

My mother was desperate to help me slim down, because she'd been a chubby girl. She'd gotten thin before marrying Dad, but eight pregnancies had padded her with an extra fifty pounds. "I gotta lose weight," she would always say. She was on a perpetual diet that never worked.

Holidays—when I would eat more than ever—were the only time when my mother would say, "Ronald, maybe you shouldn't eat so much." As Italian Americans, holidays revolved around food and family. We would spend every Easter and Christmas at Grandma and Grandpa Morelli's house a few miles away on Winthrop Street in Detroit. The house was a twenty-four-foot square, as was the basement. Down there they had a washer and drier, a stove, a fruit cellar, and a large work table for making sausage and pasta. On the other side of a cement wall was a huge table where the whole family would enjoy holiday meals.

On Christmas Eve, it was an Italian tradition to eat a dry salty fish called *baccalà*. We also had Italian wedding soup with chicken meatballs as part of the ten-course meal. Then on Christmas day, we'd be back for another feast.

Regular days at my grandparents' house were a food fest too. Grandma always kept Lorna Doones and windmill cookies inside a white Hamilton Beach roasting stand in the kitchen. All the grandchildren knew exactly where it was, and she was thrilled when we'd come over and eat.

My grandparents were very frugal. They'd lost their house during the Depression. When Grandma would buy whole chickens at the butcher, any parts that didn't get eaten at meals went into a giant pot to make stock that would be used for soup. She'd boil the carcass, head, neck, and feet. After she drained the stock, it was fun to nibble on the scraps. I remember grabbing chicken feet and sucking the meat off them as the toes spread out on my face. At the time, it didn't seem gross. It was delicious. Food in Grandma's kitchen was love, and I couldn't get enough.

But when I was eleven years old, my passion for food inspired concern in my mother's warm brown eyes, and she said, "Ronald, we're going to a doctor who can help you lose weight."

"Geez," I wondered, "why aren't I good enough as I am?" She was already taking me to tutors and summer school because my grades weren't good enough. Now my weight was another reason to feel unacceptable. Decades later, as a parent, I realized that my mother, bless her heart, wanted to do everything possible to make sure her firstborn was healthy and happy.

But at the time, I felt downright lousy.

That is, until I discovered a perk to putting on pounds: one-on-one attention from my mother. As my mom drove me to the diet doctor, we were alone in our station wagon. The backseats were empty; the car was quiet. No babies or toddlers were squirming in car seats or on siblings' laps, crying for her attention.

It was just me and Ma. And I loved it.

The doctors made me feel bad; being alone with my mom made me feel good. I had the same realization when she took me shopping in the "husky" department to buy the only clothes that would fit me—unstylish black or blue polyester pants for my school uniform. It didn't matter that we were clothes shopping—we were alone, and I felt even happier than if I were eating peanut butter.

Having an amazing Italian cook for a mother was not an ideal weight-loss situation for an adolescent food addict. If the first doctor put me on a diet, I probably stuck with it for a week, maybe two, losing a few pounds. But pretty soon I'd be devouring hefty portions of pasta and sneaking peanut butter again.

"Are you kidding me?" my mother scolded, once she discovered my hollowed-out jar trick. "Did you eat this?" She was upset that the jar looked full in the cabinet and she hadn't bought more.

So my mother took me to one doctor to "cure" my peanut butter habit. Even as a twelve-year-old, I knew the doctor was a quack. He did an allergy test on my skin to pinpoint reactions. He said I had a sensitivity to peanut butter, so he gave me a tiny bottle of peanut butter extract.

"Put a few drops of this under your tongue when the craving strikes," he said. Of course that didn't work.

I was almost thirteen at this time, and I was beginning to notice girls. But as the fat kid, I was invisible to them. "That will soon change," I told myself as I stuck to my new diet.

So I created the peanut butter diet. At first, it worked! I'd eat small amounts of it, with controlled portions of baked chicken, vegetables, and salad. It worked because I was consuming fewer calories, thanks to smaller portions.

The initial water weight melted off. But pretty soon my appetite roared back. The immediate gratification of eating was far more powerful than the far-off idea of dieting for months to become attractive to girls.

Yet I didn't understand why, if I had always wanted desperately to be thin, I had never been able to simply eat less and lose weight. The equally confusing answer was that this voice, this power, this beast, was deep inside me, telling me to stuff myself. It told me to use food to feel good, even though it made me feel so bad.

At school I'd wonder how normal-weight classmates could just stop eating when they were full. What was it like to wear clothes from the regular kids' department? What was it like to run and play with a light, mobile body? How did it feel to have your thoughts *not* be consumed by eating or the self-consciousness of being fat? My biggest wish was to reprogram my brain to think and eat like a "normal" person.

YOU TRY TO MAKE YOURSELF INVISIBLE

My self-consciousness hit an all-time peak in high school. In tenth grade, I became one of three thousand students at Southfield High School. Public school felt huge, indifferent, and scary compared to the intimate Catholic-school environment I was used to.

I hated high school. I never took my coat off. Never went to my locker. I didn't even know where it was. I loved to retreat to the bedroom I built in the basement of my parents' house. It had a pool table and a stereo. In the neighborhood, I hung out with the same guys I'd known since I was ten.

When you're heavy, you try to make yourself invisible. You walk around with this awful self-consciousness that makes your heart pound with worry that something could happen at any moment to remind you just how unacceptable you look.

That's why I never put myself in a position where people could make fun of me. I rarely went to a football or basketball game. I joined no clubs. I never had a date, never went to homecoming or prom.

"This is the hand I've been dealt," I told myself. "I am what I am, and I certainly can't twitch my nose like in *Bewitched* and change it. This is what it is."

I raised my hand *once* during high school, in English class, to talk about the racial tensions simmering in and around Detroit after the riot in 1967. Our school was mostly Jewish, with one black student.

I put as little effort as possible into academics. If I had to write a book report, I'd do it in the class before it was due.

Did I get teased?

I was occasionally called "fat." But being legally deaf in one ear probably helped me *not* hear cruel comments. A few overweight guys were teased, but they were slobs. Their hair was messy and their clothes were dirty and wrinkled.

My mother made sure that my collar was pressed, my hair was combed, and my clothes were clean.

In the lunchroom, I'd have milk and a sandwich then flee. If nobody saw me eat, then they wouldn't think I was fat, right?

FAST FOOD, FAST FAT

I weighed 352 pounds when, as a sophomore, my mother took me to my first Weight Watchers meeting.

"Ethel!" shouted the older woman who was weighing me on a scale that went up to 350. "He's too heavy! Can you get the adapter so I can weigh him?"

I wanted to disappear. No big surprise, I abandoned the program and dove back into my comfort zone: eating like there was no tomorrow.

That summer of 1969, however, I decided to lose weight once and for all. So I locked myself in my basement bedroom during times when I was tempted to eat. Rather than join the family for meals, I made up my own diet and would only eat tiny portions from a small refrigerator in my room.

My parents pretended to oblige my request to lock the basement door at night so I couldn't sneak up to the kitchen. But I know they unlocked it just as quickly so I would be able to escape if there was a fire.

I lost weight at first. But when you're addicted to a fork, and you have to use it three times a day, it's easy to lose control. I'd gain back everything I lost, and then some.

Little did I know, my food addiction was about to go haywire. The first fast-food restaurant, McDonald's, opened near our home in 1970. I was one of its best customers.

I went there in my 1966 Galaxie 500 coupe with a 352 cubic inch, four-barrel carburetor engine, dual exhaust pipes, and Mickey Thompson tires. It was black with a red interior. "Jackin' up cars," as we called it, was what I loved to do with my friends after school and on the weekends. We'd also build go-carts and mini-bikes with engines. We'd race or cruise Woodward Avenue, then later Telegraph Road.

After all, it was the Motor City, home of Henry Ford and the world's first freeway.

My hot rod put me on the fast track to morbid obesity. I just couldn't get enough hamburgers and fries under the glowing yellow arches. I'd hang out there with my buddies, who would talk about homecoming and prom. Sad that I was missing out, I'd return to McDonald's alone and order four times what I'd nibbled with my friends.

"I shouldn't be doing this," I thought while eating alone in my car. My monstrous appetite was roaring. I had no power over it; I just had to feed it, as much and as often as possible.

But at the same time, I wanted to finally control my hunger and my weight. I would never truly enjoy life, or have a girl-friend or a wife, if I kept getting fatter.

I was ready for something drastic.

I'd heard about the first intestinal bypass surgery in the late 1960s: doctors had devised a procedure to remove part of the small intestine to promote weight loss. (Today's procedures leave the organs in). I'd heard reports about people suffering horrible health problems and death after this surgery, and my mother was very upset that I would even consider it. But I was desperate.

So in 1971, I consulted a doctor, who said that at age seventeen I was too young for the surgery.

"You're never going to be thin," he said. "You're always going to be fat. If you eat twice as much as everybody else, then just eat every other day."

What a screwball!

Hopeless yet again, I just kept growing. When I graduated in 1972, I weighed four hundred pounds.

Only once did my father speak of my weight. An article in the newspaper about an eight-hundred-pound man prompted me to say, "Geez, how does that guy get around?"

"Maybe you should start thinking about that," Dad said.

I think my father stayed out of my weight problem because he knew my mother *wasn't* staying out of it.

But even her efforts to help were not enough to stop me from blowing up like a balloon. As a result, I was ordering bigger and bigger clothes from the KingSize catalog. The clothes were drab: giant dress shirts and black or blue polyester pants. I was lucky to get a decent-looking coat.

I got so big that when my buddies would invite me to the movies or to a Tigers, Lions, or Red Wings game, I'd pass. I didn't fit in the seats. After a while, they'd stop inviting me. I had a "chick magnet" car, but no chicks.

Food was my best friend and my worst enemy.

Soon after high school graduation, I did one of the dumbest things of my life: walk out of registration at Oakland Community College, about twenty miles from my parents' house. After standing in a long line leading to the crowded registration table, I learned that the only available auto mechanics' classes met very early in the morning or late in the evening. I thought about driving back and forth, and how much I'd hated high school. And I just left without registering.

Fortunately, my brother-in-law's uncle sponsored me to take classes on auto mechanics and auto sales at the General Motors Technical Center in Warren. He also helped me get hired as a mechanic at Les Stanford Chevrolet.

My life revolved around doing two things I loved: working on cars and eating.

Since I was living with my parents, every day my mom made my lunch. I ate it while driving to work. There I bought more food from "the roach coach," a truck that sold tuna sandwiches and egg-salad sandwiches, Hostess pies, pop, and other junk. It returned for lunch, and I'd eat more. In the evening, I'd go out with my buddies to chug beer and eat pizza.

My weight spiked well over four hundred pounds.

At that point, the only place I could weigh myself was the giant outdoor scale at the post office in Redford. My aunt had worked there and told me the scale went up to one thousand pounds. At night, when the post office was closed, I drove there to weigh myself.

The experience was all wrong, from start to finish. First, I was driving my cool hot rod, which should have been used for the kind of fun that young men usually enjoyed—going on dates, hanging out with friends, or going to drive-in movies. Instead I was pulling up, after dark, to the deserted post office dock.

Even though I was alone, I felt this awful sense of shame and self-consciousness. I was so heavy that I didn't dare step onto a scale for humans. And I prayed that no one would drive up and catch me in the midst of my shame. My heart was pounding so hard that I barely heard the traffic sounds from the street on the other side of the post office. Then when I stepped onto the metal pad on the scale, I watched in horror and disgust as the red dial shot past one hundred, two hundred, three hundred, and finally came to rest on four hundred pounds!

The reality of that number made me open my eyes wider and stare, to make sure it was real. At the same time, though, it was no surprise. I weighed twice what a normal man should weigh because I ate three to four times what a man should eat in a day. Harsh as it was, this reality was not powerful enough to motivate me to change. My brain's automatic response to negative feelings was to soothe myself with food. So I zoomed away from the post office, pulled into the nearest fast-food drive-through, and stuffed down all those bad feelings with a bag full of burgers and fries.

The following year, I was so disgusted with my body that I signed up for the new Optifast liquid diet at a local hospital. I thought, "Here's the magic! Here's the answer to my lifetime of struggles!" I thought this diet would change my body and my life, that I'd never struggle with weight again, and that I'd be happy.

Inspired by these visions, I consumed the nutrient-rich protein drinks. I went to the hospital several times a week for doctors to monitor my blood sugar, blood pressure, and heart rate.

I quickly lost more than 100 pounds. But as I approached 330 pounds, something happened. The possibility of being thin scared the crap out of me. As ironic as it sounds, my fat served a purpose, to literally create a comfort zone around me that shielded me from taking risks. I'd never get rejected or heartbroken if I never dated. I'd never face defeat in sports if I were too fat to play. I wouldn't have to worry about failing in a spectacular career if I felt too bad about myself to go to college. I wouldn't have to worry about being popular and being invited to ball games, concerts, or movies if I made myself too fat to sit in the seats.

Why I was so afraid, I didn't know. But this was how I had always felt. And rather than analyze that fear and get over it, I retreated back to the euphoria of eating. Those hundred-plus pounds returned fast.

Meanwhile I was promoted to car salesman. When I became too fat to fit into the cars, I sold trucks.

In 1975 I was hired at Bob Ford in Dearborn. My coworkers smoked; I started puffing through a pack or two every day.

Fatter than ever in 1977, I walked into an orthodontist's office and said, "Look, I want to lose a ton of weight, and I want to know if you can wire my teeth shut."

The orthodontist agreed. It cost a couple of hundred bucks, plus twenty dollars every week for him to remove the wires so I could brush my teeth. Then he'd wire them back.

Meanwhile, since I talked for a living as a salesman, I cut little rubber wafers out of an old football mouthpiece to hold the back of my teeth open. That way my speech sounded natural, and nobody knew that my teeth were wired shut.

I lived on gross-tasting stuff called "predigested liquid protein," which I bought at the drugstore. To prevent myself from choking if I vomited, I carried wire cutters on a string around my neck so I could cut the wires if necessary.

I thought it was okay to put my life in danger, because I was desperate to try anything. Since I'd had braces as a kid, my thinking was that if I couldn't put any food in my mouth, I'd lose weight.

After six months, I'd lost 140 pounds. At 320, the same fear of being thin roused that beastly foodaholic with a vengeance. I cut the wires off my teeth. In ninety days, I gained back all the weight, and then some. One day at a store, I ran into the dental tech from the orthodontist's office. She exclaimed, "Oh my God! We thought you died! You never came back."

"I was embarrassed," I confessed to her, "because I took the wires off myself."

Fortunately, I was doing well as a truck salesman. In 1978 I bought a house in South Lyon, a quiet suburb northwest of Detroit. But a recession hit; car sales tanked.

So I started a company with another guy and began painting apartments for a hundred dollars a day. I hated everything about it—the detail of doing the edges, the smell, the mess. Sloppy paint clothes made me feel worse about my ballooning weight.

One day when I got home from work, my mother called, "Come to the hospital, Ronald. Your father had a heart attack."

Still wearing paint-splattered clothes, I stood in the hospital hallway with my mother and siblings as they wheeled Dad past on a gurney. He waved and smiled as if nothing was wrong.

I took his resilience as a good omen for my future, especially after learning that he'd driven himself to the hospital. But Dad's health scare didn't make me think about what I was doing to my body.

I was horribly lonely. Sometimes I would go home on the weekend and not speak a single word until I returned to work on Monday.

Food became more of a best friend than ever.

I couldn't do grocery shopping for the week because I would eat until all the food was gone, usually within two days. If it was in the house, I had to eat it. If I bought lunch meat and cheese, or peanut butter and jelly, and a loaf of bread, I would just keep making sandwiches. I'd make one or two and eat them. Every fifteen minutes, another sandwich would end up in my hands, mouth, and stomach. Over and over, until the bread, meat, cheese, peanut butter, and jelly were gone.

If I bought a Boston cream pie, I'd eat the whole pie. If I made a pot of chili, with the goal of eating a serving or two each day for a week, I'd eat bowl after bowl until the pot was empty. Sometimes I would cook two pounds of ground beef, make five burgers with five buns, and devour them in one sitting. That usually happened on the couch, while watching the local and national TV news.

My craziest binge involved an entire loaf of bread made into French toast. Imagine: twenty slices of bread, six or eight eggs, milk, cinnamon, and nutmeg, all mixed together and cooked on a griddle. Then I put the French toast into a ten-by-thirteen-inch Pyrex dish, smeared it with butter, and poured on maple syrup.

I sat at the small table in my kitchen and ate it all.

Part of me believed that I liked the sensation of feeling like my stomach was about to burst, because I always ate until I reached that feeling. It mellowed me out, weighed me down, and made me so focused on the discomfort that I stopped thinking about my loneliness.

For me, this feeling was like the alcoholic who chugged drinks until he passed out. A drunk or a drug addict, however, couldn't function at a job. As a foodaholic, I could.

In 1982 my cousin and I opened a video game arcade about an hour away, in Bridgeport, Michigan. I rented out my house and converted the back of the arcade into an apartment.

Kids came to play games after school and on weekends, while I sat all day behind the counter. My meals came from the nearby Chinese restaurant, Wendy's, and McDonald's. During the four years that I owned the business, I probably gained eighty pounds. I hid under giant flannel shirts and dark polyester pants, long hair, and a bushy beard.

When you're that heavy, personal hygiene is tough. I used a shower brush with a long handle to clean under various skin flaps and folds of fat. I sweat a lot and always had to carry a hanky to mop my forehead. My pants would wear thin between the thighs from the friction when I walked.

I saw no way out of my foodaholic nightmare. When you get like that, you're almost at a point of no return. Unless you can go somewhere to lose massive amounts of weight, you don't even want to try the conventional stuff. It would take too long. You think, "Weight Watchers isn't going to do it if you're 450 and want to get down to 190." Instead you always look for that easy, fast fix.

My next fix came through the television screen, as I watched *The Phil Donahue Show*. The equivalent of a male Oprah back in the eighties, he was interviewing actor James Coco, who said he'd lost a lot of weight at a residential weight-loss facility called Structure House in Durham, North Carolina. We had no Internet back then, so I called information, got the phone number, and called. Structure House mailed me brochures, and I read every word. As I've mentioned, it cost eight hundred to one thousand dollars *every week*.

"I'm either gonna come back broke or thin," I told myself as I sold the business and my house.

I was euphoric, thinking, "This is the magic solution for all my problems!"

I was thirty years old and weighed 460 pounds when I drove to Durham the day after Christmas in 1984.

As I've mentioned, I, amazingly, soon became the star of the show at Structure House. I was losing weight faster than any person who'd ever been there. I lost fifty pounds in thirty days and then dropped one hundred pounds in ninety days.

I even got engaged! Imagine a guy who'd never had a real date or a girlfriend falling in love and discovering the joy of sex! I was excited about life and love and my future. Since sticking with the diet and exercise program felt so easy at Structure House, I was sure that I could maintain the same self-control back home as a thin guy.

Some of my greatest dreams were coming true.

And then I ran out of money.

After five months in weight-loss nirvana, I went home broke and still well over three hundred pounds. It was June 1985. I was thirty-one, living with my parents, with no job, no college degree, and no money. I drove a beat-up car. Fortunately, I got a job making a couple of hundred bucks a week moving fifty-pound sacks of flour at a food-distribution company behind a pizzeria. Soon I was delivering cheese and dough to other restaurants around metro Detroit.

Sadly, my fiancée lived in another state, and I realized that we had shared a romance of convenience, nothing more. She broke off the engagement; I buried myself in food.

The scent of baking pizza tantalized me all morning. For lunch I'd devour a whole pie, a giant meatball sub, or an antipasto salad covered with cheese, fattening meats, and oily dressing. Since I lived with my parents, I couldn't bring home a bag of five burgers for my dinner. They would say, "What the hell are you doin'?"

But I sure could eat them in my car before I got home. A short time later, I got an apartment. Many nights I would lie in bed painfully bloated.

"Please, God, help me," I cried. "What am I doing to myself?"

Then I would have the same dialogue in my head that every heavy person has had a million times: "Tomorrow I'll do better. Tomorrow I'll eat healthily. I'll stop abusing my body with food. I've dropped a hundred pounds in a couple months. I can do it again. Easy. Starting tomorrow."

Tomorrow comes. You're not nauseous and stuffed anymore. You're thinking, "Okay, I can do this." You whistle off to work.

But lunchtime comes, and you're hungry. You eat way more than you'd planned. That triggers an "all or nothing" mentality—now that you've blown the diet for the day, you might as well just eat whatever you want. So you do, especially in the evening when you're home alone. And then you're right back where you started.

Miserable. Confused about why you torture yourself. Desperate to kill your addiction before it kills you.

At least I was making progress at work. In 1985 I led a start-up company called R & P Foods, a distribution center for a local pizza franchise.

In 1986 I quit smoking—and ballooned up to 487 pounds.

The sadness in my eyes and the depressed expression on my face inspired my family to stage an intervention. My family, which worked for the same company that owned R & P Foods, convinced the owner to hold my job if I went back to Structure House to try it again.

I agreed. That was the best decision of my life, because I met Becky.

| # BECKY

Together, We'll Never Be Fat Again

I had a fluttery feeling in my stomach when I met Ron in the dining room at Structure House.

"Becky," my friend Pepper said, "this is Ron. He's from Detroit. Ron, this is Becky. She's from Atlanta."

I thought Ron was very attractive, and he had a "life of the party" charisma about him. When he shook my hand, I pretty much melted. He cast the most intense look at me, like no man had ever done. It was like his hazel/green eyes were just beaming with intrigue and adoration.

My experience with men had been the exact opposite prior to my meeting Ron: mean "fat girl" comments from classmates, cruel taunts from strangers on the beach, and awkward dates that sent me running for the Oreos and milk.

So this surprisingly hot romantic moment was a total shock. And for the first time in my life, I was in a place where my weight wasn't a source of pain and shame. I loved being one of the thinnest women in the room.

"We're playing water volleyball tonight," I said. "Do you want to play?"

"You any good?" Ron asked playfully.

"I've got a mean serve," I teased.

"Then we'd better be on the same team," Ron quipped. "I don't want to get knocked in the head and forget I met you." He smiled at me. I smiled back. And it was *on*.

That night, when I walked into the indoor pool area in my bathing suit, I didn't exactly feel like a beauty queen, but I also knew that no one would snicker or shoot a disgusted look at my fleshy stomach, hips, and legs. This loving, affirming environment felt like paradise.

Even more exciting was the hope that I was ending my lifelong battle with my huge appetite and pear-shaped body. I dreamed of weighing a slim 125 or 135. Just twenty-three years old and a year out of college, I believed so many possibilities would open up for my career, my love life, my future if I were no longer a slave to food and fat.

All this flashed through my mind as I joined Ron, Harry, Pepper, and many others in the large pool for volleyball. We laughed and splashed ourselves to an odd mix of exhaustion and exhilaration.

That night in my apartment, I couldn't sleep. Every time I closed my eyes, I kept seeing that look in Ron's eyes when he shook my hand. It made me feel like I'd been drinking champagne, and I couldn't wait until morning, when I'd see him again.

Before breakfast, we took a beautiful walk with our group through Durham's pretty neighborhoods. Birds were chirping and tulips and magnolia trees were blossoming all around the historic homes. It sounds corny, but it was the kind of thing I'd seen in movies and read about in books.

"I really believe this is it," Ron confided. "The last time I was here, two years ago, I dropped the weight, but it came right back when I got home. This time, though, I feel different. I'm going to finally lose the weight and keep it off."

I smiled. "I feel the same way." That fluttery stomach feeling that I got around Ron was the ultimate appetite suppressant. It was even better than M&M's, cheeseburgers, or cookies dunked in milk.

"Never again," I told Ron, as we headed into group therapy to analyze our food addictions. "I'm never going back to that out-of-control feeling where I want to eat every high-fat food imaginable."

"I'm with you on that," he agreed. We shared a long stare and smile that promised much more than we were ready to say.

We saw this program, and our budding relationship, as the doorway to the future we'd both always dreamed about. We were inseparable; it felt like we'd known each other forever, and the idea of ever being apart was unimaginable.

Our relationship was like speed dating since we were together so much. I'd never had that kind of intense, romantic attention, and I loved it. Something about Ron's spirit and sense of humor made me feel more at ease than I'd ever felt with anyone.

"I love the philosophy of this program," I told him over our lunch of pitas stuffed with lightly dressed bean sprouts, cucumber slices, and beets and then cantaloupe. I was referring to the orientation, when Dr. Gerard Musante had explained that he founded Structure House in 1977 to teach out-of-control eaters to use "structure" in their daily eating, to plan meals, and to learn portion control. We chose our menus for the week in advance, and cooks prepared the meals, which were served to us in the dining room.

"I'm a planner," I told Ron. "I love to organize things in notebooks and binders, and to plan menus and events."

Whenever I talked, Ron listened intently. He also had a way of engaging the other ten people who usually sat with us at mealtimes.

We followed the diet perfectly. For dinner we might have a four-ounce beef burger patty with fat-free cheese on a piece of bread or a grilled chicken breast with half a baked potato or summer squash, and then fruit. At every meal, a beverage bar offered iced tea and water but no carbonated or caffeinated drinks.

Our bodies were shrinking rapidly. Some of our peers would sneak off to the local mall and indulge in french fries dipped in mayonnaise. But not us. Bitten by the love bug, we wanted to look and feel our best.

"Becky, I want to know everything about you," Ron said. "Absolutely everything."

MY LIFE WAS HAMBURGERS

I was six years old and just as tickled as a girl could be. Standing in front of the three-way mirror in the dressing room of Belk's Department Store in Decatur, Georgia, I twirled and smiled in a little two-piece turquoise flowered bathing suit with yellow trim. I felt so pretty and happy.

Until I looked at the sales clerk.

Her face twisted in a look that let me know that I was anything but cute.

"Girls your size don't wear suits like that," she snipped. She handed me a suit with a loose-fitting baby doll top and ruffles. With one disapproving glance, that sales clerk scarred my self-esteem and body image for life. It made me want to hide my body and conceal the huge appetite that had made me chubby and ashamed for as long as I could remember.

Born on July 2, 1964, I grew up near Atlanta, Georgia. My dad was an obstetrician/gynecologist at a university, so he worked long hours at his office and at the hospital. He and my mother, a registered nurse, met at a hospital in Atlanta. After they married, Dad's work in the navy took them for a while to Guantánamo Bay, where my brother was born. He is six years older than me, and my sister is two years older than me.

We lived in a small bungalow in a middle-class neighborhood, and Mom stayed home to take care of us. One day, when I was five, my parents sat me down at the table and told me I was adopted. My mother said, "Somebody asked us if we wanted a baby." My childish imagination envisioned complete strangers knocking on the door and saying, "Here's a baby, do you want it?"

It took me several years to figure out what adoption meant. Yet I never felt that my parents loved me any less than they loved my brother, who was their biological son, or my sister, who had been adopted as well.

When it came to food, though, I was very different from my normal-weight siblings. They had an enviable detachment from food: when they were full, or when the cookie was eaten, they were off to the next activity. Period.

Me? I wanted to eat as much as my stomach would hold, and then some. I thought I was born with an "eat everything gene." My four-hundred-pound father was the same way. Would I someday grow up to be that big? Why did I love eating so much?

Our family ate dinner together every night. Mom made everything from scratch, serving balanced meals that always included a green vegetable and another vegetable, like corn, and a lot of red meat. I especially loved it when she made these little ground steak burgers wrapped with a piece of bacon. Casseroles were a staple at our dinner table. Every southern casserole has two mandatory ingredients: sour cream and a can of creamed soup, such as mushroom, celery, or chicken. She'd mix in meat, noodles, and peas, then top it with crumbled potato chips, crackers, or bread crumbs. It was the ultimate home-cooked comfort food before anybody thought of calling it that. And I couldn't get enough. But when I'd try to scoop up a second or third serving, she would say, "You don't need any more of this. Why don't you have more vegetables?" Portion control seemed so easy for my mother, who was very thin and had a light appetite.

She never told me, "Girls aren't supposed to eat a lot." I simply understood that if you're feminine and ladylike, you don't overeat—it's not pretty. I also understood that it was different for boys. I would hear neighbors and family friends talk about their teenage boys who could eat them out of house and home, and that was not only acceptable but even a badge of honor.

For me, being a girl with what felt like a teenage boy's appetite, it was the opposite: shame. If one piece of pizza was good— two or three or more were even better. If a small milkshake would hit the spot, then a large one was better. It was all about more. While my brother, sister, and mother seemed to have an automatic ability to stop eating when full, I didn't, and it showed.

In school pictures, I was heavy looking but not obese. Throughout my childhood, I was active, but that didn't make me slim down. When I wasn't bouncing on the trampoline with my brother and sister in the backyard, I played fullback on my public school's soccer team. I also played softball in the spring.

Still, I was embarrassingly out of shape. And it wasn't even in gym that I became sadly aware of this. It was during a family vacation, a time when kids are supposed to be carefree and have fun.

Not me. We were vacationing with my mother's sister on Jekyll Island and all running on a gravel road. I couldn't believe it when my aunt, my mother, and my cousins blew past me. I was so disappointed with myself. It seemed weird that a kid couldn't run faster than the grown-ups. If only I could have loved exercise as much as I loved food.

With my friends, I always ate more than anyone. Once, when I was ten, I spent the night at my best friend's house, and we made homemade waffles for breakfast.

"Oh my gosh!" she said. "Nobody could ever eat a whole waffle. Not even you."

But I was thinking, "I want more because I could eat this easily." That moment made me feel bad, as if I should feel embarrassed for wanting to eat the whole waffle. After seeing fat kids teased at school and in public, especially if they were eating fattening food, I had a very clear understanding that I would be looked down on if people saw how much I really wanted to eat. That made me want to hide my eating. Oddly, even though people could see my plump body—the evidence of my secret eating—I never wanted to confirm the cause by overeating in front of them.

In seventh grade, my embarrassment turned to shame and downright pain. We had to move to Philadelphia because my dad got a yearlong fellowship at the University of Pennsylvania. It was a horrible year for me.

We rented a condo in a complex where several of my classmates lived, including some of the cool and popular kids. I wanted to fit in so badly, but I never did. Instead kids made fun of me because I was fat.

I think my home economics teacher felt so sorry for me that she gave me the Good Citizenship Award during a ceremony at the end of the year. I was sure she thought, "Here's this fat girl with a southern accent in the middle of Philly."

I felt lonely while walking through the hallways, sitting in class, and eating by myself in the cafeteria. This made me wish

I were invisible, so nobody could ignore me or spew a "fat girl" insult.

One of the worst experiences was when all the kids got weighed in gym class. I was just paralyzed with dread that I would have to step onto a scale in front of all those boys and girls. I was certain that I would be the laughing stock of the school. Gym class was always a source of stress. In the locker room, we had to change into our gym uniform—shorts and a T-shirt—in front of the other girls. I remember trying to hide while changing clothes, so my classmates wouldn't see my chubby body. We also had to swim as part of gym—which of course meant wearing a bathing suit. I dreaded this and hated every minute of standing on the pool deck waiting for someone to say something mean about my fat body.

Whether boys and girls tried to whisper their insults or said them loud enough for me to hear, I heard it all.

"She's chunky," a girl would whisper in the locker room.

"Thunder thighs," a guy would smirk in the hallway. It was horrible when it happened, but the fear of when it would happen next, as I walked to class or ate lunch, was just as bad.

After school, nothing comforted me more than M&M's, cookies, and ice cream. I had a sweet tooth the size of Texas, and I was never happier than when I was satisfying it.

Fortunately, we moved back to Atlanta a year later. During our weeklong drive from Pennsylvania to Georgia, I set a goal: for every meal except breakfast, I would eat a hamburger or cheeseburger, with fries. As we were driving, I entertained myself by wondering, "What version of a hamburger am I gonna eat?"

Other times, when we ate out, I didn't base my order on what might taste best. My criterion was which dish would give me the most food.

The great pleasure I felt while eating caused an equal amount of emotional pain in school.

"Fatso!" a boy would say, disguised under a cough, as I walked to the chalkboard to answer a question for the teacher. His buddies would laugh as I stood at the board with my wide backside on full display.

The same thing happened when I entered classrooms for my "job" as an office messenger. If I had to take a note to a teacher, or get a kid out of class to come to the office, I would tense with dread as I opened the classroom door. I would brace myself for someone to make a "fat girl" comment as I entered. Too often, they did.

At the beginning of eighth grade, I was horrified to hear another girl say that we were going to the "weight room." I had no idea that meant weight lifting as part of gym class. My mind was racing a million miles an hour. How could I get out of this? What would happen when I stepped on the scale in front of the boys and the thin, pretty girls in my class? I was so relieved to arrive at the weight room and realize I would be spared the humiliation of standing on a scale in front of my classmates!

A short time later, even though I was never confident with boys, I invited an overweight boy to the Sadie Hawkins dance in eighth grade. I wore blue jeans, a striped blouse, a denim vest, and brown shoes.

We started with dinner at Pizza Hut. I ate a slice or two, and I wanted much more of the delicious pizza on our table. But I told myself, "You shouldn't eat a lot when you're on a date."

I felt more awkward as the night continued. Inside the school gym was a pretend train with little boxcars that had straw on the floor. Kids were buying tickets to go inside and make out. I went in with this boy, and kissing him was horrible. I freaked out.

"Mom," I pleaded into the phone that the teacher chaperones

had let me use well before the dance was over. "Please come get me. I want to go home. Now!"

I didn't feel better until I was home with a plate of Oreo cookies that I dunked in milk. This made me feel safe and comforted for a while. But the resulting fat caused more misery.

That summer I was thirteen and walking on the beach during our vacation with family friends in Jacksonville, Florida. I was wearing a green one-piece bathing suit with a yellow stripe up the side. I had just stopped wearing the more concealing baby-doll-style suit. Out of nowhere, a guy, a complete stranger, taunted, "Why don't you lose fifty pounds and call me in a week?" Devastated, I felt like a whale on the beach.

Why would people who didn't even know me make such a sport out of commenting about my body? They didn't care that my name was Becky or that I was smart and planned to go to college. All they saw was the evidence of my huge appetite, which their cruelty only made worse. I probably put on weight to hide from people like that jerk on the beach, but the bigger I got, the more of a target I became.

THE YO-YO DIETING BEGINS

In high school, I had two best friends. One was naturally thin; the other was chunky like me.

At lunchtime we'd sit in the cafeteria, and I'd wish I could have my thin friend's nonchalant attitude toward food. She'd eat whatever she wanted, just enough to feel full. End of story. I would marvel at her with envy, wondering how I could be that detached from eating. But I couldn't.

I felt emotionally connected to every bite on my tray. I always bought the same lunch: a tuna-salad sandwich laden with real mayonnaise, potato chips, milk, and a Little Debbie oatmeal cookie. I savored every bite and wished for more when it was all gone. But I was so self-conscious about eating in front of other people, I didn't dare eat a bite more than what looked like a "normal" lunch.

My constant shame about wanting to eat intensified my desire to eat in secret. When I was alone, I was free to savor the flavors of cookies or candy without the critical or scornful stares of others.

Even though I felt pretty down about myself, I tried to project a positive appearance. I never hid in big, sloppy clothes. Instead I dressed really nicely to make up for my imperfect body. During the late seventies and early eighties, the preppy style was in. I had a closet full of chinos, Pappagallo belts, and espadrilles. I was so into my wardrobe that I made a chart listing what I would wear, so I wouldn't repeat an outfit.

The problem was that the cute clothes at popular stores like the Limited didn't fit me. They went up to size 14; I was at least a 16. But I would have died before I let anyone see me walk into a plus-size store like Lane Bryant. So I devised all kinds of ploys to hide the truth about where I shopped. First, I would walk past the store to make sure I didn't see anybody I knew. Then I would duck inside, always careful to make sure no familiar faces were entering to expose my secret.

I wouldn't write "Lane Bryant" in the check register. I had a code name for it, so even if my friends ever saw my checkbook, they would never know where I'd gotten the cute skirt and sweater they'd just complimented.

At one point in high school, my best friend and I decided that we would lose weight once and for all.

Our parents paid for us to do the Nutrisystem diet. The program provided prepackaged food, and we had to attend support group meetings. We were so excited! We couldn't stop talking about how we would get slim and cute, and wear all the coolest clothes.

Posters of skinny, blonde, smiling Farrah Fawcett were all the rage during that time. The TV show *Charlie's Angels*—with three thin, pretty female detectives—was also popular.

Thin was in. Chubby was not. At all. Striving for these impossible standards of beauty kept me and my friend eating salads, baked chicken, and the prepackaged Nutrisystem foods for a few weeks at best. Our cravings for cheeseburgers and fries, and ice cream and cupcakes, were even stronger. All the fun of eating our favorite, fattening foods doomed the Nutrisystem plan to a growing list of failed diets. Whatever weight we lost, we gained right back, and then some.

We also tried Weight Watchers. We were the youngest girls at the meetings. The older women were very nice, but it was hard for us to follow the diet. And getting weighed at meetings, with everybody announcing how much they'd lost or gained, was just awful. I'd feel so ashamed that I would go home and eat more.

After I got my driver's license, I loved being able to secretly stop at stores and buy sweets. But I realized it wasn't so secret— or fun.

Once, I had just driven to a Dunkin' Donuts and was walking up to the door.

"Do you *really* need that?" yelled some teenage girls who were getting into their car.

Crying, I got back into my car and went home without buying doughnuts.

I hated that I wanted to stuff myself with junk, but I never found the power within myself to eat healthy meals with smaller portions so that I would feel and look better. In fact, I had an "all or nothing" mentality about eating. Either I was strictly following a diet down to every calorie or I was bingeing on fattening food. Chronic dieters are always either losing or gaining. I didn't know how to enjoy balance and the middle ground. I became a yo-yo dieter. Losing weight, gaining weight, up, down, up, down— like a yo-yo.

My weight stayed up over two hundred pounds when I went to the University of South Carolina. I was far from home, with no friends, living in a dorm with a roommate from Florida who spent all her time on the phone with her boyfriend.

I, on the other hand, had no boyfriend—not even any prospects on campus. As for food, I still hated eating in front of people. I always felt ashamed, as if I should feel bad for being hungry and wanting to eat. If my roommate was away, I could easily eat a whole pizza, alone in our room. The dorm had a twenty-four-hour cafeteria, and I was no stranger to cheeseburgers and pizza. I also couldn't get enough Bojangles' chicken. No surprise, I gained the freshman fifteen and then some.

"I'm not happy here," I told my parents over the phone. "I want to do something else."

"Why don't you go to Emory?" they asked. After all, both they and my sister had attended the university in Atlanta.

The following year, I lived in a cool little apartment with my friend from high school—the one who had attended Weight Watchers with me—in a pretty part of town with old houses. I had friends, and I even joined the Alpha Chi Omega sorority. It was nice to have a social life and meet new friends. But I never attended the fraternity parties. The few dates I had usually ended badly, and I'd soothe my hurt feelings with Oreos and milk. Even though I dressed neatly and liked to wear cute outfits, I didn't think I was attractive enough for any guy to see past my weight and like me enough to date me.

With my friends, I ate a lot of pizza. By myself, I made frequent stops at the Wendy's drive-through during the five-minute trip home to see my parents. Alone in the car was the perfect place to eat. No one would see me or judge me, and I was free to enjoy the delicious flavors without guilt or shame.

Especially cinnamon-raisin biscuits from Hardee's. Two came in an order, and they were drenched with white sugar icing. They were amazing. I'd also get sausage biscuits, and I was in heaven for those few minutes.

I didn't try to eat healthily or set goals to lose weight in college. I wished I were thin, but I didn't know how to make it happen. I never tried to exercise by joining a gym or taking a walk.

Someday I wanted to marry and have kids, but I had no real vision for life after college. When I graduated in the spring of 1986, first I worked at Rich's department store in the Liz Claiborne department; then I worked as a recruiter at a headhunting agency for doctors. I hated making cold calls. I was very awkward and wasn't good at it.

One day I was talking with my supervisor about the employee party we were planning. I got really animated, gesturing with my hands, offering creative ideas for the food and the decor.

"Becky, I really wish you'd be as excited about your job as you are about this party," my supervisor said.

So there I was: an overweight twentysomething who hated her job. Then my doctor said my high cholesterol could kill me. It was over 500.

I had to change but didn't know how. Then I saw a TV commercial about Structure House. I called my dad at the hospital where he worked and asked him if he would have lunch with me in the hospital's cafeteria. He must have known I had something big to talk about because I had never done that before. But I wanted to talk to him alone because I thought that he—

weighing four hundred pounds—would understand why this was so important to me.

Also, I needed to ask him for financial help to go to Structure House. I'm sure that he went home (or back to his office) and immediately filled in my mom about my request. They agreed to let me go—meaning that I would have to quit my job and move away. My mom and I went up to visit Structure House. Encouraged by the staff and facility, we hoped that this would be the answer for me. I felt strongly that my parents would have done whatever they could to help me lose weight.

Little did I know that I was about to fall in love and feel better about myself and my life than I had ever imagined.

CHAPTER **RON AND BECKY**

A Future as Sweet as Candy

RON
I'd Never Felt Happier

We have a photograph that was taken at the Structure House Halloween party. Becky and I are dressed up like giant bags of M&M's. I'm wearing a yellow package with brown words for Peanut M&M's. Becky is wearing a huge brown sheath that says "M&M's Plain Chocolate Candies" in white letters. We're both smiling in the photo, because we were thrilled to think that we'd always have each other to help us live healthier and keep off the weight.

It was amazing to fall in love in that spa-type atmosphere. We felt a million miles away from the real-world pressures of working, paying bills, and managing hectic schedules. All we had to do was to follow the program and lose weight.

"We'll never let each other gain weight again," Becky said one day, while we were driving around Durham and looking at pretty houses. "We know the struggles, and if one of us is falling back into our old habits, the other one will be there to stop it. So we'll never be fat again."

We were inseparable, until Becky went home for her brother's wedding. When she returned to Structure House, she moved into the apartment beside mine. We fed a twenty-five-foot telephone cord from her apartment into my place by drilling a hole in the wall! That way, when Becky's parents called, she could answer as if she were in her apartment.

After about four months together, I had to return to my job in Michigan.

We said good-bye in the parking lot before I drove back to Detroit. Years later I would find out that Becky went upstairs to her apartment, grabbed her purse, and bought ingredients for chocolate-dipped Oreos. She thought that would make her feel better, but after the euphoria of indulging, the guilt and nausea only made her feel worse.

When I returned to visit, it was like a scene from a romantic movie when Becky jumped up to hug me. That "lost in love" feeling was still the best appetite suppressant ever.

A short time later, we got into my car and hit the road for Atlanta. We were going to tell Becky's parents that she was moving to Michigan with me. Thankfully, her parents gave us their blessing. They weren't thrilled about her moving to Detroit, but they could see that she was thin and happy, so they accepted our decision.

This was in November of 1987. We moved into my apartment, in a growing upscale suburb of Detroit, and I felt like the luckiest guy in the world. Becky and I got along so well—we even worked together. While I handled the distribution of cheese, pizza dough, and other ingredients for the pizzerias served by R & P Foods, she worked as an office assistant.

As for eating, we were on Structure House autopilot. Becky had brought home the menu cards to plan our meals for the week, and she'd shop for vegetables, fruits, and low-fat meats to prepare our healthy meals. I was so impressed; she even assembled binders full of low-calorie recipes.

The companionship that we shared every day, and the sense of teaming up to keep our food demons at bay, was amazing.

At Christmastime, Becky experienced the family and food extravaganza at my parents' house. They were thrilled that I was in love, and they welcomed Becky into the family.

Somehow, despite the Italian feasts on holidays, we got back on track with healthy eating. In fact, even though we worked around pizza and subs all day, we would go out to lunch for healthy fare like salads with grilled chicken. We'd even bring our own low-fat salad dressing, a trick we'd learned in Durham to save hundreds of calories.

The weather was not a pleasant adjustment for Becky. Her only experience with frigid temperatures, icy roads, and snow was during her awful year in seventh grade in Philadelphia. But she tolerated the Michigan winter because, she said, being in love in the North was better than being lonely in the South.

I was about to make it even more worth her while. One day in January, we went to dinner at Mountain Jack's, an upscale steakhouse near our apartment. We were at table 604, and I had conspired with the staff to bring a bottle of wine to accompany my surprise after dinner. But I couldn't wait.

"Becky, will you marry me?"

"Yes!"

We were the happiest people ever as we celebrated with wine, salad, steak, and baked potatoes—butter and sour cream on the side, of course.

BECKY
My Wedding Dress Was Tight

Happy moments like that, with food as a celebration of love, began to expand our waistlines. We were both working full time and planning the wedding. Suddenly, the stress of real life returned.

First, my father lost feeling in his legs. I went to Atlanta for his spinal surgery, after which he used a wheelchair.

Then, back in Michigan, a temporary job agency placed me at GMAC, handling leases for the financing arm of General Motors. That became a full-time job.

Meanwhile, I was planning the menu, the music, the flowers, the program, and gift baskets that Ron's family members would find in their hotel rooms in Atlanta. I was also being fitted for a dress. It had long lace sleeves, a fitted taffeta bodice with a sparkly lace overlay, and a full skirt with a five-foot train. I felt so beautiful and excited when I first tried it on. After all those years of being lonely and called "fatso" in school, I was actually getting married. But during the first fitting, the waist on my wedding dress pinched my stomach. And I burst into tears.

Most brides try to lose weight for the happiest day of their lives. Me? I was blowing back up.

Worried about Dad and dealing with the stress of a new job and our upcoming wedding, I had soothed my nerves with Oreos and milk more than a few times.

Creeping back into our old eating habits and gaining weight happened slowly, over many months. Ron and I gradually abandoned our calorie-saving tricks. We'd use full-fat salad dressing at lunchtime, or Ron would bring home a "test pizza," or we'd go to dinner and not ask for the sour cream and butter on the side for the baked potato. An extra 300 calories here and 600 there really added up.

Gradual weight gain doesn't hit you until your clothes suddenly become tighter. And nothing could be worse for a woman than a too-tight wedding dress.

On October 8, 1988, we married in Grace United Method-
ist Church, and my parents escorted me down the aisle, with
my mother pushing my father in his wheelchair. I didn't feel
euphoric. The celebration jangled my nerves. I'm very much a
planner, and it was stressful to plan a wedding in Atlanta from
Michigan. It was overwhelming to plan the rehearsal dinner,
an "out-of-towners' dinner" and a laser light show at Stone
Mountain, which is a giant slab of granite sticking out of the
ground. But we pulled it all together, and it was beautiful.
Ron was handsome and proud in his black tuxedo. At our
reception on the top floor of the State of Georgia Building,
we look ecstatic in pictures as we feed each other pieces of our
three-tiered, flower-covered white wedding cake. Our wedding dance was to the song "What a Wonderful World" by
Louis Armstrong.

We honeymooned at Las Brisas Hotel and Resort in Acapulco,
Mexico. We had a private swimming pool with a balcony overlooking the water and pink hibiscus blossoms everywhere. We chose
that resort because we could enjoy the pool without anybody
looking at us in swimsuits. We swam, lounged, ate delicious food,
watched the sunsets, and had an amazing time.

Back home we succumbed to "newlywed spread"—the typical weight that people gain when they're married. No longer on
the dating scene, newlyweds get comfortable, enjoying life by
eating out, eating in, and not obsessing about how they look.

But we aren't typical people. We're foodaholics. And when
two foodaholics fall off the wagon together, they become enablers
for each other. We'd long forgotten that conversation in Durham
about how we'd never let each other get fat again.

We were having so much fun, eating in restaurants while taking spur-of-the-moment weekend trips. We'd drive off to places

like Niagara Falls, with no reservations. It was hilarious, because we'd end up in these honeymoon motels with theme rooms. Once, we stayed in a "jungle room" full of big stuffed lions, with mirrors everywhere and giraffes coming out of the ceiling. We laughed, went sightseeing, and ate whatever we wanted.

Another time, during a weekend trip to Gatlinburg, Tennessee, I found a place to rent a romantic cabin in the woods. It had a heart-shaped fireplace and a waterbed. As soon as I lay down on the waterbed, Ron jumped on.

I was catapulted off the bed! His weight had displaced the water, and the bed had bounced me like a trampoline. We just laughed and laughed.

And best of all, we ate without any inhibitions. I was back to enjoying my childhood passion for burgers, fries, and cookies. Ron was eating anything—and everything. Even though we were "closet eaters," we weren't afraid to eat in front of each other. We saw the pounds creeping back on, but neither of us said a thing about Structure House or getting back on track.

That conversation just didn't happen. Either it was too hard, or neither of us wanted to create a conflict, or we were both enjoying the freedom of eating again.

As a result, unhealthy habits became our "new normal." I loved to dip a spoon into big bowls of ice cream at night while watching TV, while Ron ate peanut butter or lunch meats rolled up with cheese. For dinner, we'd get Chinese takeout and eat on the couch in our apartment, while watching TV. For a while, we went through a mashed potatoes phase during which we ate them every day.

Pretty soon I was back up to 210, my starting weight at Structure House, and Ron was pushing way past 400.

We were big, but we were still in love.

RON
Small Problems, Big Disasters

After saving for years, Becky and I took our dream trip: a cruise to Alaska. We were so excited as we waited for our flight from Detroit to Vancouver. All our plus-size clothes were packed in our luggage, which we would pick up at customs in Canada. But the flight was canceled. The airline put us on another plane to Seattle. We arrived; our luggage did not.

A normal-weight person would be annoyed, but he could always go buy an outfit or two to wear until the luggage showed up. A four-hundred-pound man and a size 20 woman cannot. "All we have is what we're wearing!" Becky cried.

The slim airline guy tried to console us: "Oh, Mr. Morelli, I know how you feel."

"Look at us!" I shouted. "Are we supposed to go to the Gap and start sewing things together? There's nothing on the ship that will fit us."

To add insult to injury, they put us on a tiny, twenty-seat prop plane where the other passengers looked at me like, "Oh, geez, I hope the fat guy doesn't sit next to me." Becky hates to fly, so she was panicky for the whole flight.

Thankfully, our clothing disaster ended on the ship. Our luggage was waiting in our room, having taken another flight to Alaska.

A cruise, with its twenty-four-hour buffets, might seem like a foodaholic's paradise. But not for a closet eater. I was very self-conscious about how much I ate in front of other passengers. Eating "less" for me, however, still meant eating far more than a normal man.

I would tell myself, "I can get a handle on this. I lost fifteen pounds in my first week at Structure House. These thirty, forty, fifty pounds will come right off when I put my mind to it. I'll start tomorrow."

But tomorrow never came. I justified our eating by thinking, "I'm happy now. I have a beautiful wife. I don't care if she's as big as this house. I love my wife, and I want her to be happy. If neither of us complains about our weight, it's because we're happy with the way things are going, and we're happy with our life."

Especially on trips like our cruise.

When I saw a guy in running shorts heading for the workout room, I asked Becky, "Why the hell would you go on a cruise and work out in the gym?"

She laughed, because even though she forced herself to take aerobics class several times a week back home, she hated to exercise as much as I did.

BECKY
Pregnancy Packs on the Pounds

When I got pregnant, I was already fat again. When you're thin and pregnant, it's cute. When you're fat and pregnant, it's not cute at all. It's horrible. People can't tell you're pregnant; it just looks like you're getting fatter. Plus, maternity clothes are made for thin women with a big stomach, so they didn't fit me. Since I had to look professional while working in the GMAC office, I bought bigger clothes at plus-size stores.

But I was thrilled when my doctor said that I could skip aerobics during the pregnancy.

Ron and I were ecstatic about becoming parents. As two people who'd been lonely and sad, we were creating our own version of the American dream. We were even building a new house in South Lyon. With its historic downtown, the sleepy suburb was the perfect place to raise children.

I loved eating for two! So much so, that I gained forty pounds. At the same time, however, Ron was probably eating for three or four. The promises we'd made at Structure House remained forgotten as we focused on cribs, furniture, and paint for the nursery.

Especially when we panicked with the realization that, two weeks before the baby was due, our two-story, white colonial had no drywall.

"Give me the keys to your house," Ron told our builder, "because if my wife has this baby before the house is done, we're moving in with you." I even faked a contraction at the closing, all in fun. We moved into our home just in time to welcome seven-pound, eight-ounce Michael into the world on May 5, 1990.

I stayed home full time. Most new moms want to lose weight, but the fatigue, the crying, the diapers, and the nighttime feedings make it hard enough to take a shower, much less prepare a salad. When Ron was at work, I'd push Michael around the neighborhood in a stroller. But I was still eating whatever I wanted.

"When are you due?" someone asked.

I was horrified. Because I wasn't pregnant. I was just fat. Then, twenty months after Michael was born, we were blessed with eight-pound, four-ounce Max on January 13, 1992.

After two pregnancies, I was my biggest ever: 260 pounds. I was constantly thinking, "I have to lose weight. I have two babies—it's time to slim back down."

But that never happened. Instead we launched into the busy pace of family life.

RON
Fiending for Fast Food

While Becky was home with the babies, I'd go to the Wendy's drive-through for lunch. I'd get three double cheeseburgers, a spicy chicken sandwich, four large Cokes, four large fries, and I'd supersize everything. I'd pretend to read from a list, as if I were picking up lunch for the office staff. But I'd eat it all in my car, then return to work, where I'd sit at my desk. I was secretly eating 7,000 calories every day and getting no exercise.

By the time Max was born, I was huge, weighing in at more than five hundred pounds.

My size didn't stop us from traveling often. It was easiest to drive, with the boys in car seats while Becky and I were comfortable in the front seats of the SUV. We'd drive to Atlanta to visit the grandparents or to the North Carolina shore to rent a condo on the beach.

When we did fly, it was a grim reminder of life as a fat person in a thin person's world.

Imagine a crowded airport. A 260-pound mom and a 500-pound dad are pushing a double stroller loaded with two crying boys and two bulging diaper bags. We're each carrying a car seat. Every time we pass a gate, people give us this horrified look, like, "Oh my God, don't stop here!"

The scornful stares only got worse on the plane. As we'd squeeze down the aisle with our babies and gear, passengers would glare again, because nobody wanted to sit next to the fat person with a crying baby. We solved that problem by each sitting next to one of the boys, who were strapped into car seats on the airplane seats.

The most humiliating thing about flying, however, was

asking for the seat-belt extender. While looking into the flight attendant's face to ask for it, you just want to disappear. You sweat. Your heart pounds. You hope nobody hears and snickers.

Plus, those seats are torturous for big people. The fat on our backs and butts pushes us forward, giving us even less legroom. You pray the guy ahead of you doesn't lean his seat back and crush your knees. Lower the tray to drink or eat? Forget about it. It would never go down over our bellies.

For the whole flight, you wish that one day you'll be able to fly as a thin person. No stares. No embarrassment. No seat-belt extender.

For my fortieth birthday, I was diagnosed with diabetes and sleep apnea, which makes you suddenly stop breathing while you're asleep. It's a huge problem for obese people. I would have already been dead if our family physician, Dr. Michael Balon, had not diagnosed me in 1992. He recommended me as one of the first patients in the sleep lab.

"You're the worst patient we've ever tested," the staff said after videotaping me for a night in a double bed. I laughed so I didn't cry, as I watched myself stop breathing 370 times, including once for ninety seconds.

"I'm so sorry," I told Becky.

"Some nights I would stare at you," she said, "wondering if you'd start breathing again."

The doctor gave me a sleep apnea machine, which includes a face mask that looks like something out of science fiction but forces me to keep breathing through the night. The day after I first used it I realized, "Oh my God! I can't believe this is how the rest of the world sleeps. I'm never taking the mask off!"

Within eighteen months, my doctor put me on medication for hypertension and high blood pressure. I thought, "I weigh more than five hundred pounds, I have two little babies, and my body's starting to fall apart. Something drastic has to happen 'cause this ain't gonna work. Now what?"

The answer: gastric bypass surgery. The procedure was new then, back in the mid-1990s. No hospitals were doing it. So we researched it for a year, getting opinions from different doctors. Would it be safe or make me even sicker?

BECKY
The Shame and Secrecy of Fat

As Michael and Max became old enough to feed themselves, I served foods that they would eat, especially macaroni and cheese, pasta, breaded chicken, chicken tenders, and frozen entrées like lasagna. Unfortunately, I was not thinking about calories, fat, or what the healthiest choice would be for two growing boys. I didn't want our children to have the shame or bad feelings that I felt while eating as a child. I wanted to make mealtime a fun, happy experience for our family. And that meant serving foods that would not elicit complaints from the boys—make them whine or refuse to eat. I wanted to feel that we had the perfect family, and that by keeping everyone happy at the dinner table the boys would automatically eat "normal" and never endure the pain that Ron and I felt.

In hindsight, Ron and I were very naive to think that our children would not mimic our penchant for huge portions and fattening food choices. During many intense conversations about how to deal with our children's diet and weight, we had decided that we would never make a big deal about what our boys ate or how much they weighed. We felt that our parents' efforts to help us eat less and slim down had only made us feel worse and eat more. We believed our laissez-faire approach would keep them normal and slim.

In truth, we had a happy home life. We'd play in the yard, or the kids would help with gardening. We have lots of photographs of the boys just being silly, playing with each other or goofing around with us. One photo shows me wearing denim shorts and hugging four-year-old Max in the kitchen while six-year-old Michael tugs his arm. We're all grinning.

One special thing I did every year was to let my creative passion for baking go wild when it came time to make the boys' birthday cakes. Creating sweet treats was a way for me to express love as a mom, and the boys appreciated every bite! One picture shows birthday boy Max sitting with Michael and other kids at the dining room table. They're all smiling around a white platter holding a frosted brown rectangular cake adorned with dump trucks, trees, Peanut M&M's for rocks, and miniature plastic people beside a big candle in the shape of the number five.

Despite all the fun, I was really worried about Ron's weight. I hoped that bariatric surgery would work. Even though the doctor told us about the potential risks—like excessive bleeding or even dying—we were desperate, because he was really suffering. That filled me with worry and sadness; not only was my weight ballooning, but I was terrified that our sons would lose their dad at an early age and I would be a widow. I feared that Ron was eating himself to death.

We have a framed photograph of Ron and the boys in our family room that speaks to the pain—and unspoken shame— behind Ron's smiles.

It shows him wearing a black turtleneck and trousers, kneeling behind the boys. Four-year-old Max has bowl-cut blond hair and a big smile, while six-year-old Michael has the same haircut and grin. Both boys are wearing jeans and white turtlenecks. They're adorable; Ron looks proud.

But many years later, Ron confessed that his knee was hurting so badly during the photo session that he said, "Just take the damn picture." His knee was so traumatized from balancing all that weight that he could barely walk for a week.

"The next day," he said, "I went to get my car's oil changed, and I slipped in the garage. I could not get up! I actually had to wrap my arms around the car hoist. The workers pressed a button to raise it, and I held on."

Ron was living with so much embarrassment and shame about his weight that he just couldn't speak about the obvious— not even with me. He was hurting, physically and emotionally, and he needed help.

RON
I'll Never Have to Diet Again

In August 1995, I checked into the Bariatric Treatment Center about ninety minutes southwest of Detroit. At 527 pounds, I was terrified that I would die on the operating table. Would the three-foot incision over my huge gut—from my breastbone to my groin—kill me?

I was terrified that Becky would have to raise five-year-old Michael and three-year-old Max by herself. That's why, for the day of the surgery, I insisted that my parents sit with her in the waiting room. If the doctors came out to say that I was dead, at least she wouldn't be alone. As grim as this sounds, the alternative was to continue committing slow suicide with food. There's a reason it's called "morbid" obesity. It kills.

Before going in, I showed Becky all the important papers

pertaining to insurance and bank accounts, in case she became a widow.

During the four days prior to surgery, I was not allowed to eat. My stomach and intestines were supposed to be empty. Drinking juice and water, I spent a lot of time hugging Becky and the boys, and praying that I would survive the surgery to spend a long life as a thin man with my family.

It was worth the risk if I'd finally win my lifelong battle with food and fat. I thought, "I'll finally be a normal size. It's one big, easy fix, and I'll never have to diet again."

"After surgery, your body won't tolerate fatty foods or sugary foods," the doctor told me. "Eating too much sugar will cause nausea. Too much fat will cause uncontrollable diarrhea."

"Boy, that's a blessing," I thought, "being physically unable to eat the junk that got me this way."

On the day of the surgery, I was horrified when the nurses put a breathing tube down my throat while I was conscious. They explained that this was typically done after a patient was put to sleep with anesthesia. However, the anesthesiologist said that if they put me to sleep and then pressure from my weight prevented them from putting the breathing tube down my throat, they would be unable to perform the surgery or give me oxygen if something went wrong. Despite the numbing drug they sprayed on my throat, I gagged something horrible.

Thankfully, after that my surgery went smoothly. I had a procedure called Roux-en-Y gastric bypass.

Doctors sliced away a small portion of the top of my stomach, and then stitched it up to form a small pouch. Meanwhile, a hundred centimeters of the lower portion of the small intestine, which connects with the colon, is snipped and connected to the new stomach pouch. Not only does this restrict the amount of food that the stomach can hold, but it stops absorption of calories in the shortened small intestine, where calorie absorption occurs.

My prayers were answered: I survived the procedure. My stomach was now the size of an egg, and the opening to my small intestine was as small as a pencil eraser and initially even smaller because it was swollen. At first I could only take a few sips of liquid. After a couple weeks of consuming only clear liquids, the opening healed to the size of an M&M. I progressed to pudding, Jell-O, and pureed foods. I put steamed vegetables, lean meats, and beans into the food processor to make them like baby food.

After six weeks, I could eat solid food, such as chili or sloppy joes. But if I failed to finely chew my food, I'd cough, run to the sink, and spit it out.

Meanwhile, I was losing weight so fast that I became the leader of my bariatric surgery support group. About twenty men and women—who were either considering the surgery or had already had it—would gather to talk about the procedure, the side effects, the worries, and the excitement. While I did not attend prior to my surgery, going to the meetings afterward enabled me to share an intoxicating sense of hope and excitement that helped us all feel that we would finally get thin and live the full, happy lives we'd dreamed about. The support group was also a safe place to talk about gross things such as uncontrollable diarrhea if we ate certain foods (for me it was dairy products; if I ate them, I'd better find a bathroom within three minutes!). Others expressed worry about what they would do at a wedding dinner or how they would resume normal activities like shopping if they were feeling nauseous, vomiting, or having diarrhea.

We also shared recipes. Since we had to puree everything we ate, some patients actually ate baby food. Me? My old habits roared back with a vengeance: just three or four weeks after

surgery, I told the group something that became legendary fodder for future support groups: "I pureed a Big Mac!"

It was cold, mushy, and bad, so I threw it out. I only told Becky
about it later, because I was afraid she'd wonder why I would do
something so crazy. Meanwhile, I felt comfortable enough with
my support group to confess that the fast-food junkie within me
was still fiending for drive-through junk. And that kept me constantly pushing the limits on what I could eat. I discovered I could
hold down part of a McDonald's Filet-O-Fish if I pulled off the
bun, wiped off the tartar sauce, and just ate the flaky white fish
in the middle.

Five or six weeks after my surgery, doctors began removing the staples from my three-foot-long incision. After they had
removed about a third of the staples, they realized that I had not
healed enough, so they left the remaining staples in my skin.

Imagine my horror when, a short time later, the incision
split open! The opening was a foot long, two inches wide, and
an inch deep! It wasn't bleeding; it looked like a slice through
raw steak.

I was frantic, thinking, "Oh my God! It's gonna split open
more and my guts are gonna fall out!" Becky was ready to pass out,
but she composed herself enough to drive me to the local hospital
emergency room. The ER doctor used surgical tape to seal the
incision, and it healed just fine.

The support group played an important role for me, especially
when sharing the gory details of that drama. Everyone was going
through physical and mental changes that the average person
wouldn't understand, so it was comforting to close the door and
talk about embarrassing or uncomfortable topics.

Meanwhile, I was still eating very little, and in less than a year
I had lost nearly two hundred pounds.

My success inspired Becky to have the procedure eleven months after me. I teased her that she waited to make sure it didn't kill me before she did it herself.

BECKY
I Was Thrilled for Both of Us

As a woman who believes that "you can never be too thin," I had surgery to lose weight for my looks. I'd like to say I was motivated by high cholesterol after my cardiologist said losing weight would be healthier for me. But the truth was that, at my top weight of 260 pounds, I was tired of looking and feeling bad. Max was in preschool; Michael was in first grade. I wanted more energy to keep up with their busy schedules, and I wanted to set a better example for them in the kitchen.

Like Ron, I hoped this was the magic solution to finally kill my huge appetite. If my stomach couldn't tolerate cupcakes and cheeseburgers, then I would stay thin forever, right?

That's what I told myself as they sedated me to surgically alter my stomach. Ron's parents kept the boys during my procedure and the early part of my recovery. It was painful, especially if I coughed or moved. And I developed a hernia that needed repair a year later.

It was hard at first to figure out what I could eat. Once, at Red Lobster, I ate a shrimp and a scallop and was stuffed. At home I ate tiny portions of lean meats and vegetables. I loved feeling like I'd finally found a solution to losing weight and keeping it off. It seemed like 125 pounds just melted off my body.

Ron and I had taken huge risks to have surgery, and it paid off: we both felt and looked amazing.

RON
My Most Disgusting Surgery Ever

Thanks to weight loss after my bypass surgery, my huge gut had deflated, leaving a three-foot "apron" of skin hanging to my knees. So I had surgery to remove the excess skin. During the procedure, an upside-down T incision extended from my solar plexus to a line between my hip bones. It took 1,256 stitches to close it, leaving a tubelike hollow that I had to pack with gauze twice a day. It was disgusting; I was glad I could do it myself by looking in the mirror so Becky wouldn't have to pull out forty feet of bloody, gunky gauze from my gut. Every day I needed less gauze, which was covered with less bloody gunk. After six months, it finally healed. Boy, was I thrilled to have a flat stomach!

After the surgery, I weighed 318—the lowest since my early teens. I was off medications for diabetes and high blood pressure, thanks to losing so much weight. But when they removed the skin I also lost so much blood that I became anemic. A few weeks after the surgery, I felt horrible. My doctor sent me to the hospital, where they pumped me with fluids and blood.

For the first time since Structure House—a whole decade before—Becky and I were both thin. This accomplishment ushered in a golden era for our family life.

When the kids came downstairs one Christmas morning, they found a big, stuffed Mickey Mouse in the middle of the floor.

"What's that?" asked Michael.

"Yeah, what's that for?" demanded Max.

"We're going to Disney World!" I announced.

"When?" the boys asked.

"Right now!" cheered Becky, who had planned the trip.

The bags were already packed and waiting in the car, as were the dogs, who had a reservation to stay at a kennel during our weeklong trip to Florida. Four hours later, we were at Disney World.

As we explored the Magic Kingdom, Becky felt and looked great in her slim denim jeans. It was easier for me to walk. The boys—husky but not fat—stayed energized on ice cream, chicken fingers, fries and burgers, and pop. With the fattening treats came worries that our children might pack on extra pounds. But when weight has caused so much pain in your life, you just don't want to think about it while your family is at Disney World.

Or on the cruise we took to the Bahamas. We have a great family photo of us by the ship's railing (it's a fake backdrop). Becky is slim and smiling in a sleeveless floral-print dress. I'm relatively small, in a brown suit and tie. But the boys are definitely husky. We had no idea that within a matter of years both Michael and Max would be morbidly obese, second-generation foodaholics.

Take a peek into our photo albums, and you can literally watch us become a fat family. And if you hold two particular photos side by side, you'll see just how quickly that happened.

I had a jaw-dropping moment recently when I looked at the family photo of us on a Caribbean cruise after Ron and I had surgery. We were both slim and happy looking, and the boys were a little chubby but not markedly overweight. The shocker came when I compared that photo with the shot of us on a family vacation just a year later in Las Vegas. I did a double take and thought, "Whoa!"

Eight-year-old Max and ten-year-old Michael appear to have gained a significant amount of weight since the cruise photo. I look plumper too, posing with the boys on a huge boulder in Red Rock Canyon.

Yes, I was gaining weight, and so was Ron. Even after successful bariatric surgeries, Ron and I were really struggling. A french fry here. A cookie there. A cupcake, a bite of pizza, a burger . . .

We were horrified and delighted to discover that our egg-size stomachs would tolerate increasingly larger portions of these allegedly taboo foods. By "grazing," or eating small amounts all day long, we could eat quite a bit.

Now, if you're wondering how in the world Becky and Ron could actually gain weight, with egg-size stomachs, well, here's what they *don't* tell you before bariatric surgery: that little opening between your stomach and small intestine stretches. When the tiny stomach fills up, and you keep eating, the food gets pushed into the small intestine, which holds more food.

Ron could still eat a couple of burgers. I could easily eat a big salad. And once a foodaholic discovers that "I can eat fattening foods again," it's nothing but trouble.

Especially during a family vacation, when we relaxed the rules even more and ate as much as we could. That Las Vegas trip was a blast, and eating made it even better. We rented a Chrysler Sebring convertible, dark charcoal with a red interior. Driving through the sunny Nevada desert was adventurous. Lunch on the road? Burgers and fries for all of us. Of course we'd stocked up on snacks for our excursion: beef jerky, Combos, M&M's, and Pringles.

"Dad, do we get to go back to the hotel buffet for dinner?" Michael asked as we returned to the Mandalay Bay Resort and Casino.

"We'll be there within the hour," Ron answered as he navigated the highway.

"After dinner, we'll take a swim," I said.

"Cool!" the boys cheered as their handheld video games chirped.

Back at the hotel, we stood in the long, winding line for the restaurant buffet. It reminded us of those mazelike lines at the Cedar Point Amusement Park in Sandusky, Ohio.

But for the Morellis, the buffet was the ultimate amusement—a lighted maze offering every food imaginable.

I wanted to try everything, and then go back for more of what was good. Ron and I could eat a lot but not nearly as much as before our surgeries. I hated thinking, "People are staring at the fat family like we're gonna rampage the buffet."

The boys were ready to eat their way from one end of the buffet to the other.

Ron piled his plate with roast beef, shrimp, pasta, rice, and nachos. I couldn't resist a burger with salad and a dinner roll with butter. We could take only a few bites of each item. But the boys went wild with mac 'n' cheese, fried fish, burgers, and fries.

Then we all sat down in the enormous, bustling dining room, among countless families and waiters bringing refills of pop and water, and the noise of silverware clanking on plates. All around us was laughter and the other sounds of families having fun on vacation.

Sllluurrrpp. Max made that loud sound when his straw sucked up the last droplets under his ice cubes. He giggled; we all laughed.

"I'm so thirsty," Max said. "The desert made my throat feel like sawdust."

"We're putting this buffet to shame," Michael said, devouring his second plate.

Max nodded as he bit into his burger.

"This prime rib melts in your mouth," Ron said, returning to the table with another plate.

Why didn't anyone stop this dinnertime indulgence?

Because when you're on a family vacation, you want to enjoy it. Nobody would have a good time if Mom or Dad were nagging about eating vegetables instead of fries or salad instead of burgers.

Besides, when Mom and Dad were eating anything and everything, we couldn't very well tell the kids to do differently. Kids learn from what they see. And we had been horrible teachers from the moment they'd opened their eyes.

Even worse, strangers cast disapproving stares, especially at the pool. As we walked out on the huge patio, stopping at the cabana for towels, guests looked at Ron, who wore a white T-shirt with his swim trunks. Then they looked at two mini versions of Ron. In their swim trunks, the boys had big bellies and chubby chests.

Watching Ron and the boys splash into the water, as people stared in disgusted fascination, reminded me of when I was a girl, hearing mean comments as I walked into classrooms or on the beach.

I hated that we had become a fat family whose next generation was vulnerable to ridicule. I cringed at the thought of our children being teased and feeling bad.

But somehow when you sit down to eat, you escape into the pleasure of food and forget the pain of fat.

"We shouldn't be eating like this," my conscience told me. It wasn't right for us to eat with such wild abandon. Dinner was just a replay of our breakfast feast of bacon, eggs, sausage, pancakes, waffles, and French toast.

Vacation was simply a supersize version of our foodaholic lifestyle at home. And here at the all-you-can-eat buffet, what better way to top it off than with a piece of chocolate cake to soothe Mom's anxiety as the boys made towering ice cream creations at the sundae bar.

"I shouldn't be letting them eat like this," I thought. "It's not good for them to eat thousands of calories at every meal."

The slice of cake looked rich, with thick layers of frosting on top and in the middle. I loved the feeling of my fork pressing through the piece near the skinny tip, catching a nice swirl of frosting. I put it in my mouth, and . . .

Heaven on a fork. It was delicious beyond words. Lost in the pleasure of this double-chocolate flavor fest, I thought of nothing but the joy of sweetness in my mouth.

SKINNY WIFE, FAT FATHER, CHUBBY BOYS

Days, weeks, and months were whizzing past as our bad eating habits made us all fatter and fatter. It was devastating that Ron was gaining it all back after a huge weight loss *for the fifth time.*

Yet in the midst of this, I did something neither of us had been able to do: Stop.

It happened in 2001, a few years after the Las Vegas trip. I was working a part-time job at Edward's Cafe and Caterer in nearby Northville. Ron was now vice president at R & P Foods.

I loved working the counter at the quaint, upscale café. It was popular for chicken potpies, chicken and broccoli salad, cherry chicken salad, pasta salads, and brownies.

I'd leave work in time to pick up the boys from school, then take them to Cub Scouts or sports practices. Sometimes we would go home and do things like bake chocolate chip cookies.

"How long will it take, Mom?" Michael asked as I put the first cookie sheet in the oven.

"Five to seven minutes," I said.

"I want milk with mine," Max added.

I ate some raw batter, savoring the gooey sweetness and crunchy chocolate chips while thinking, "I shouldn't be eating this. But it's so good. I'll just have one cookie, and tomorrow I'll get back on track with salad and grilled chicken. I'll drop these extra pounds and . . . No, you won't."

Michael and Max laughed as they clanged their spoons into the batter bowl. Chocolate chips fell to the floor, where our dogs, Salvatore and Sophia, scrambled to lick them up.

It was an all-American scene that any mother would love: two happy boys having fun with their mom and the dogs in a nice suburban home, after a full day at private school, while Dad worked.

But my boys were fat.

And it was my fault.

Our fault. Ron and I had inflicted our foodaholic ways on them, and they were growing up to be just like us. On the counter sat a yellow envelope of pictures we'd developed from recent trips to Florida and the North Carolina shore. On the beach in their swim trunks, Michael and Max both have bellies and chubby chests. One picture shows Max fishing on a boat. He's holding a fishing pole and a fish that he caught, and his belly is on full display. Another picture shows Michael posing by the water in shorts and a T-shirt that does nothing to hide what would look like a pregnancy "bump" on a woman. I hate pictures of myself if I look fat; seeing "fat pictures" of our kids made me want to cry.

How could we have been so naive as to think that they wouldn't follow our bad example? And how could we stop it?

No! Something inside me snapped. I never wanted them to feel as ugly and unacceptable as I had felt in the dressing room at age six in that cute little bathing suit.

I had to show them a better way so they wouldn't end up weighing four hundred or five hundred pounds like their dad.

"Mom, are the cookies almost ready?" Michael asked, his round face glowing with anticipation.

Max set three glasses on the counter and got the milk from the fridge. "I'm pouring a glass for you too, Mom."

I mussed his hair and looked at him and Michael like they were the most beautiful children on the planet. No matter what, all I wanted was to keep them this happy.

So I didn't have the heart to say that we shouldn't eat cookies today. That we should go for a walk instead. And that when we returned, I would make a lower-calorie dinner instead of the pizza Ron would bring home or the cheesy, beefy lasagna that I had already prepared and stored in the refrigerator for dinner.

Instead I wanted to keep the smiles on my sons' faces as we munched the homemade cookies. When that buttery, warm cookie full of melted chocolate oozed into my mouth, it was so delicious that I lost myself in the taste and texture. For a moment, the pleasure quieted that guilty voice in my head.

"We want more, Mom," the boys said.

"No, it's almost time for dinner," I answered.

"But it'll take so long for you to bake the lasagna," Max said. "We won't let it spoil dinner. We promise."

"Please?!" they pleaded.

Before I knew it, they were helping themselves to more cookies.

"Tomorrow," I promised myself, "I'll be more forceful in saying no. Tomorrow I'll serve a less-fattening dinner."

The cookies made me feel fat. I was afraid to put on my jeans because I knew they'd feel tight in the waist.

"You're gonna get really fat again . . .

"All that effort—including surgery!—and you still can't keep the weight off . . .

"Once a fat girl, always a fat girl . . .

"No!" I felt like a switch flipped in my head. It wasn't magical. It wasn't like music played. It was hard to change the way I thought about food and even harder to discipline myself to eat healthier meals and fewer calories. What would I do instead of eat to comfort myself? Because every time I looked at my increasingly overweight children, I felt a horrible guilt that made we want to lose myself in ice cream and cookies.

But somehow my newfound determination to finally over-come my self-inflicted torture with food and fat made me get a grip and stick to a plan. It really was like a switch flipped on inside me, and my motivation surged to an all-time high. I devised a strict food plan for Monday through Friday. On the weekends, I enjoyed higher calorie foods, in moderation. *This* is the big magic secret to losing weight and keeping it off. It's all about calories. I counted them religiously. And I burned them, with morning Jazzercise and evening walks around the neighborhood. Over the next year, this regimen helped me drop the thirty pounds I'd gained after surgery.

I had reached a point where nothing could get me off track. I desperately wanted my family to join me. But without Ron's support, it was impossible.

"What's for dinner, Mom?" asked twelve-year-old Michael. "It sure smells good." He stood beside me as I opened the oven.

"Mmm-mmm," I said. A hot gust of garlicky herbs hit us as we peeked in at a Pyrex dish containing golden brown chicken breasts.

"Perfect," I exclaimed, donning oven mitts to put the chicken on the island beside the big salad bowl, mixed vegetables, and red skin potatoes.

"Mom," Michael protested. "We want something good, please."

"Spaghetti and meatballs!" said ten-year-old Max.

"Sorry, guys, this is what I made tonight, for all of us."

As I took plates from the cabinet, we heard the garage door rumbling open.

"Dad's home!" the boys cheered, bolting down the front hall to greet him. I could hear them turn the corner as Ron opened the door.

"Yea!" the boys cheered. "Pizza! Breadsticks!"

In the kitchen, I exhaled angrily. How could I make the boys eat a healthy dinner if Ron was sabotaging my efforts?

"Hi, honey," he said happily as he walked in and kissed my cheek. He was carrying two huge pizza boxes topped with a smaller one that no doubt had breadsticks covered in melted mozzarella.

"I made a healthy dinner for the boys," I said, casting a disapproving look as he moved the salad bowl and vegetables to make room for the pizzas.

"We want pizza!" Max said.

"Meat lover's, right, Dad?" Michael asked.

"Yeah," Ron answered, "it's a test pizza. They used a different brand of sausage that's a little spicier but sweet too."

I rolled my eyes. Spicy or sweet, it was all fattening. My husband obviously loved the food so much that he couldn't see, or didn't want to see, what he was doing to our boys.

Or to himself. Why didn't the rows of medicine bottles on our dresser upstairs give him a clue that he was committing slow suicide? I was terrified that someday I'd have to raise two boys alone.

"I don't like spicy," Max protested.

"Don't worry, big guy," Ron said, "I brought a regular meat lover's just in case you don't like it."

I wanted to explode at him for encouraging them to eat like this. But as the boxes flew open and the boys took slices, with cheese stretching and bits of bacon glistening amid greasy circles of pepperoni and chunks of sausage, I knew it was hopeless.

It felt like we had put our sons on a runaway train that was reeling into the same nightmare of food and fat that Ron and I had been trapped in for most of our lives.

Somehow, by the grace of God, I had escaped. How could I put the brakes on what I feared would be a lifetime ride toward obesity for Michael and Max?

"I had a hankering for this all day," Ron said, loading his plate with three pieces.

"These breadsticks are awesome!" Max exclaimed, pulling off a glob of cheese that had slid onto the bottom of the grease-soaked cardboard box.

In my mind I yelled, "Cut!" as if this were a scene I could just stop. But Ron and I had already scripted this story. I needed to revise the script in midproduction. But how?

"Where's the marinara sauce?" Michael asked, finding it just as quickly in the corner of the breadsticks box. He eagerly dunked a cheesy breadstick into it.

That little plastic tub of tomato sauce was as close to a vegetable as my kids would get that night, like most nights. Here's where we'd fallen into another bad habit as a family. We'd abandoned the dinner table. Instead we'd migrated to the other side of a waist-high wall, to the two couches in the family room. Each of us had a spot where we'd eat and watch TV. The couches are perpendicular to each other; the space between them is the walkway to the kitchen. Ron sat next to the walkway at the end of one couch, with either Michael or Max on the other end, both facing the built-in shelves and television. I sat on the other couch, next to the walkway, usually lying down if we were watching TV. That couch faces the coffee table, a big chair, and a door leading to our sunroom, which contains a large table and chairs used for holiday meals. The big chair is one spot where the boys loved to sit and eat dinner.

Perhaps we moved away from the table because it was more fun to watch TV while we ate. Or maybe I just didn't want to "see" what was happening to my family as I stuck to my regimen to keep those 125 pounds off for good.

On too many nights before this, I would have been joining

in the fun, sampling the test pizza, commenting on the flavors of the new sausage, and loving every bit of bacon.

But now I was looking at our life through a very sober lens. The boys were like mini versions of Ron. Even Max's blond hair had turned dark like Michael's and Ron's hair. And they were all stuffing down thousands of calories worth of cheese, grease, and dough.

I wanted to cry. My mind was racing, searching for a solution. So I ate my 300-calorie dinner of baked, skinless chicken breast, a ping-pong-ball-size potato, and salad with nonfat dressing. As usual I sprayed I Can't Believe It's Not Butter onto my vegetables.

"There she goes, guys," Ron joked. "I can't believe it's not really butter. Help! Get me some real butter!"

The boys laughed. "It looks like light yellow spray paint," Michael teased, holding another slice over his plate. "It doesn't melt. It drips."

"It has zero calories," I said in self-defense, "and it tastes like butter."

As they took second and third helpings, I should have stood up and shouted, "We have to stop! We can't let them keep eating like this or they'll be obese like you! They'll be diabetic, with bad knees, like you!"

But I didn't have the guts. Ron was their dad. I didn't want to make him feel worse. I knew that would only make him eat more. And I especially didn't want to make the boys feel bad about themselves.

So I forked up some more salad and prayed that someday, somehow, the boys would take my side at dinnertime.

I stood up and said, "I need to take my walk before it gets dark."

I won't pretend that it was easy. While I wished I were unwrapping a candy bar, I laced up my gym shoes. While I wished I were crunching down on sweet, smooth chocolate, my feet hit the sidewalk. And I walked off my anger, my guilt. With every step, I still wished I were on the couch, eating ice cream. But my thighs were no longer rubbing together. I wasn't out of breath as I walked briskly. My blubbery stomach was gone and wasn't jiggling with every step.

My jeans were loose.

I felt skinny.

And that was the best feeling of all, for a split second. But I couldn't fully enjoy my success, because the family that I loved more than anything in life was still inside, on the couches, getting fatter and unhealthier by the minute.

In 2003 I was promoted to sous-chef, then catering manager. I loved preparing creative meals for the café and catering company. But working full time made it easy to succumb to the speed and convenience of fast food for the boys.

Especially when I picked them up from sports practice and they were hungry with hours of homework to do.

"We're hungry, Mom," eleven-year-old Max said, his cheeks red from running during soccer practice.

"I haven't eaten since lunch," Michael added. "And we have to go to the store for the stuff I need for my science project. It's due tomorrow."

In a matter of minutes, they'd be eating burgers, fries, and chicken nuggets. I felt guilty, but I knew they wouldn't want the grilled chicken and vegetables that I planned to eat at home for dinner. Ron would probably pick something up on the way home too.

On other nights, all four of us would go out to a sit-down restaurant like Red Lobster or to the South Lyon Hotel. The hotel is in a historic building in South Lyon's quaint, old-fashioned downtown, and the restaurant's menu boasts pizza, burgers, and other kids' favorites. Wherever we went, the boys would eat huge portions of fattening, greasy foods, while I picked at a salad.

So basically, at this point, whether it was from convenience or sheer defeat, I stopped cooking for my family, and the boys' weights continued to spike. The higher the numbers on the scale rose, the more guilty and hopeless I felt.

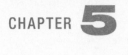

RON

Sick and Sad without My Eating Buddy

It was a Friday afternoon in early 2004. The pain shooting up from my hip felt like someone was blasting it with a blowtorch.

"Oh, geez," I moaned as I sat at my desk at Quality Chain Distribution, also known as QCD Food Service, a distribution company that I started in early 2002 after leaving R & P Foods in 2001. Little did I know, this pain was ushering in a new era of problems that would force me to face the huge financial, professional, emotional, and physical toll of my food addiction. I was literally about to reach a breaking point that plunged me into the darkest period of my life.

But I was too busy running my business to see it coming.

"Ron, we're ready for you." An employee waved for me to join my team in the warehouse to talk about inventory and distribution. Someone had already arranged the pallets and crates for me to sit as we talked.

Sitting there hurt too, but I pushed through the pain to give delivery instructions. I needed surgery, but leaving my company for two weeks to recover seemed risky. I had a great team, but Ron Morelli was the face of the company. And with two boys in private school—thirteen-year-old Michael was in eighth grade and Max was in sixth grade—this was no time to take a financial risk.

So I kept working and postponing surgery to replace the hip that had literally worn out under hundreds of pounds of fat for so many decades.

I would turn fifty soon, and I was a master foodaholic. One of our strongest traits must be denial. We do anything but face the truth. Reality hurts so much that we just don't let ourselves face it. As soon as I would start to think, "Oh my God, my boys are really putting on weight," or "If I keep abusing my body like this, it's gonna kill me," I'd numb the onslaught of worry and guilt with double cheeseburgers and fries. I stuffed down my feelings, and the aftermath of feeling lousy and bloated distracted me even more. All day, every day, for most of my life.

But now fat was literally crippling me. Never mind that I was back on pills for high blood pressure, hypertension, and high cholesterol. I was even injecting myself with 50 units of insulin, which is a huge amount. I stored the insulin in a small refrigerator in the bedroom. Every morning I'd fill a syringe and inject myself in the chest. Then I'd go downstairs and have breakfast. I gave myself another shot in the evening.

Despite all this, I had to keep my company going. I was also appointed to the South Lyon City Council, which was exciting but added even more to my plate.

Family time was also a high priority: Becky and I loved to have the boys' undivided attention over dinner at restaurants, so each Friday I'd pick them up and take them out.

"That's real attractive, Becky," I said sarcastically, hating that her blouse flaunted her collarbones.

"Thank you," she snapped back. She was as disciplined as ever, even though she worked around food all day.

I hated that we had veered in opposite directions when it came to weight. She was succeeding where I had always failed. She was skinny; I was fat. She controlled every calorie that went into her mouth; I was still hitting the drive-throughs multiple times a day. She shot out of bed before dawn to exercise; it pained me to move. She was determined never to be fat again; I had given up on myself.

I got the feeling that she wouldn't be throwing me a surprise party for my fiftieth birthday in a few months.

I had lost my best eating buddy, but I had gained two new ones: Mike and Max.

On Fridays, we usually went to the South Lyon Hotel.

"Good evening, everybody!" One of our favorite waitresses escorted us to a table. We'd been going there so long that she knew to put us in a cozy, nonsmoking corner where I could sit far back from the table and not block an aisle. When you have a huge belly, you can't sit in a booth or close to the table in a chair.

My hip was excruciating. As much as I dreaded surgery, I was eager to get it behind me and, hopefully, no longer be tortured by this pain twenty-four hours a day, seven days a week.

Sitting in the restaurant, thinking about food and ordering a delicious meal, enabled me to indulge my favorite distraction from any negative feelings. But this time the excitement of eating out was dulled by worries about surgery and finances as well as by Becky's super-picky behavior. It was a constantly irritating reminder that I was out of control and had lost my eating buddy.

She cast a serious look across the table as the boys perused the menu. She said, "Michael, why don't you order a salad with grilled chicken breast."

In typical teenage fashion, Michael looked at his mom like she'd told him to order poison.

"I'll have fried chicken and more fried chicken," he answered. He weighed 230, and Max wasn't far behind.

"No, let's get the fish and chips," Max said, "like we always do."

"Okay," Michael said.

When the waitress arrived, Becky ordered first.

"I'll have the grilled whitefish prepared dry. No oil, no butter, and no tartar sauce. Just a slice of lemon on the side. And I'd like the vegetable medley, with no butter. For my salad, no cheese and nonfat vinaigrette on the side."

The boys and I shared an annoyed look, knowing that when Becky's order arrived it would be wrong and she would send it back. That always happened. She was no fun anymore.

"I'll have the porterhouse steak, baked potato, and salad," I told the waitress.

"I'll take the all-you-can-eat fish and chips, please," Michael said.

"Me too, and more Sprite, please," Max added.

Sure enough, Becky grimaced when her fish arrived with a slight sheen of oil.

"Take this back, please," she said. "I ordered it with no oil or butter."

Meanwhile, my steak was delicious and the boys enjoyed their battered fish and fries. As we ate, I couldn't help but think, "Like father, like sons." I hate to admit it, but on one level I felt comforted by the fact that our sons had replaced Becky as my eating buddies. Yet every time I looked at what it was doing to their bodies, it scared the hell out of me. It would be my worst nightmare for my sons to repeat this horrible cycle.

HIP SURGERY THREATENS TO CRIPPLE OUR FINANCES

The pain in my hip finally became unbearable, so my surgery was scheduled in spring 2004. I reluctantly made arrangements for my employees to handle affairs at the office while I recovered; I was terrified that something would go wrong that would require my attention, and that we might lose business if it weren't handled properly.

I had bounced back from major surgery in the past, so I was confident that this recovery would be no different. Sure enough, the surgery was successful. Doctors told me to stay away from work for three to four weeks so that the eight-inch incision over my new titanium and porcelain joint would heal properly. "Piece of cake," I thought. But as the weeks dragged on, staying home to convalesce while worrying about my business became unbearable.

So I went back to work after only two weeks. What harm could it do to sit at my desk? I thought it was no big deal. Besides, I'd always prided myself on toughing it out through colds so I could get the job done and keep business booming. This time I was thrilled to be back at work, sure that my hip would heal and all that pain would be a thing of the past.

Boy, was I wrong.

"Ron! There's a pool of blood under your chair!" an employee exclaimed as he entered my office.

I immediately went to the doctor, only to learn that the incision was infected. That puddle under my chair at work was from blood and fluid leaking from the incision, which had split open.

My doctor explained that during my hip replacement, surgeons had cut through six or seven inches of fat to reach the muscle and bone. After replacing the joint, they sewed up the muscle, but you can't stitch fat very well. Think of a steak. You can stitch the meat, but the fat is like jelly. So they stitched up the skin and the jelly. But while sitting at work the arm of my chair had rubbed against the incision, aggravating it to the point of bursting.

"If this infection gets worse and goes down to the bone," my doctor warned, "you could lose your leg."

That scared me into following his directions this time. I had to stay home and rest—attached to an IV drip of antibiotics. Every four hours, for five weeks, I changed the bag to deliver a fresh dose of medication. That meant setting the alarm clock to wake me up during the night so I could add a fresh IV bag.

Becky made sure I stayed in bed or on the couch, to avoid putting pressure on my hip. At one point, my mom and Becky were screaming in each of my ears about taking better care of myself.

"If you lose your leg," Becky snapped, "what's a four-hundred-pound-plus, one-legged, fifty-year-old guy gonna do? Nothing!"

As it was, a full arsenal of drugs was keeping me going. Our bedroom looked like a pharmacy. For diabetes, I took Glucotrol and Metformin twice a day and Avandia once. My blood sugar was in the 300s—really high—before I got on the meds, which reduced it to 170 or 180. The ideal is 75–110. One Lipitor pill every day lowered my cholesterol from 260.

For high blood pressure, I took Adalat and Procardia once a day and Cozaar twice. My blood pressure stayed around 165/90, which was still high. And I also took Prilosec twice a day to calm my stomach's ulcers and bleeding.

Even with my $20 insurance copay for prescriptions, I was spending $250 a month for medication. And despite my great Blue Cross coverage, I'd probably spent $100,000 over my lifetime for weight-related medications, surgeries, and weight-loss efforts.

Because of vitamin and nutrient deficiencies after gastric bypass surgery, I still take a multivitamin twice a day. And every six months, I get intravenous iron injections at a local cancer center.

All this while sleeping with the mask connected to my sleep apnea machine, to keep me breathing through the night.

The aftermath of my hip surgery made me face the fact that my health was in crisis. It was depressing to spend the next eight months at home to heal my hip and save my leg. "It is what it is," I told myself, accepting that this was the hand I'd been dealt.

The boys never said anything, but I could see in their eyes that they were worried about my health.

"How's it goin', Dad?" they'd ask after school.

"Slowly but surely," I'd say, putting on as happy a face as I could muster.

But they looked worried when I returned to the hospital twice for doctors to open the incision, remove dead tissue, and sew it back up. This was yet another grotesque price I paid for being a foodaholic.

And just as I feared, it cost me my business. I could not run my company from the couch at home. I had great guys working with me, but I needed to be physically in the office to make it work.

No amount of peanut butter or cheeseburgers could soothe the worst anxiety I'd ever felt. Would we lose the house? How would I pay the boys' tuition? Becky was working at the catering company, but her salary alone wasn't enough to support our lifestyle.

Michael was now a freshman at Detroit Catholic Central High School, and Max would join him in two years. Then college . . .

"God, please help me!" All I could do was pray that I had the skills to start another company as soon as I could work again.

This was the worst period of my life. Fat had debilitated me. It threatened to handicap me. And it could ultimately bankrupt me.

Every time I looked at skinny Becky eating her steamed vegetables and Egg Beaters for dinner, before dashing out for a walk, I felt even worse. She was the Energizer Bunny, and I was the sickly couch potato. One night I was watching TV and snacking on deli meat.

"Who will be the Biggest Loser?" the announcer asked as heavy people appeared on the screen. I was captivated as the announcer described the new show on NBC.

"Boy, that would be great," I thought. "Go on a TV show and lose a bunch of weight." But I could barely walk, much less exercise in a gym like the contestants on the commercial. All I could do was sit on my couch, hooked up to my IV pole, and fantasize about life as "thin Ron."

As for those three little guys on the peanut butter jar, their expressions were eerily prophetic regarding my love-hate relationship with food. One guy looks angry, the middle boy looks angelic, and the third kid is licking his lips. How odd that they appeared on the label of my favorite childhood treat, expressing emotions that I would not understand for years. But, boy! Were they accurate!

These thoughts crossed my mind in October 2004 as I snacked on peanut butter and tuned in for the first episode of *The Biggest Loser*. I watched every minute. I had never related to anyone on TV the way I empathized with the contestants as they struggled to lose weight.

"I really need to change," I'd think while watching the show every week. "If they can do it, I can do it." But I never did.

Being sedentary all day, alone in the house, while Becky was at work and the boys were at school, only made it easier to eat away my sense of failure and pack on more pounds.

I felt like the biggest loser, for all the wrong reasons.

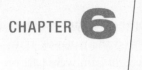

CHAPTER **6** / **MIKE**
We Ate Enormous Portions

Embarrassment. Shame. Disgust.

Those became prominent themes as soon as I got old enough to realize that what I thought was such a great life had some serious flaws.

All I saw was the positive until I was about ten. I had two loving parents, a brother who was my buddy, and a huge extended family who adored me. We lived in a nice house in a safe neighborhood. I went to private school, where I got good grades and had a lot of friends. I was a Cub Scout. And our family took great vacations.

But unfortunately, you can grow up thinking you've got a great life, and that the parents you wanted to emulate were awesome in every way, and then approach adolescence and get slapped with a bigger view of the world. You realize that what you thought was so great—being big—is really bad.

Pride turns to a punishing sense of shame.

Embarrassment becomes a constant, torturous emotion. Still, as a kid, you're not able to get all deep and analytical about it. This is your life, what you know, how things are. As my dad always says, it is what it is. It's ingrained in you, and even though you realize you don't like certain aspects of it, you're in it until you're old enough to change it.

One major moment of realization happened when I was thirteen. By then there was no way I could stop the runaway train of my appetite. Enormous portions and weight gain were part of who I was. No matter how embarrassed I felt.

Here's what happened. One night, when our family went out to dinner, I saw the receipt for the all-you-can-eat fish and chips that Max and I usually ordered. The waitress had typed into the computer: "Two orders of fish and chips. Seven refills. Yeah, I'm serious."

I stared at the receipt, my cheeks burning with embarrassment as I sat at the table with my parents and Max. I said nothing; I was just sitting there like I'd been slammed in the chest. The comment made me feel like a freak, someone who was so far off the charts that I was fodder for jokes.

On one level, I knew it was obnoxious to eat that much, at least from a "normal" person's perspective on eating (eat one portion, maybe two, and then stop when full).

But the grim reality was that Max and I ate enormous portions all the time. It was normal. It was how we grew up. And suddenly stopping, and eating only a fraction of what we were used to, well, that just wasn't going to happen.

But as I stared at that receipt, I hated feeling like my behavior was so shocking and disgusting to the waitress. In my mind, it was as if her comment grew to represent a chorus of disapproval from the whole world. And when you're thirteen, you want to fit in. You want people to like you and think you're cool, not think you're a glutton.

As we prepared to leave the table that night, all I could think was, "Holy crap. This is so embarrassing."

I hoped no one else saw the comment, and I don't know if

my parents did. I never mentioned it to them or anyone. Talking about it, even to my family, would be even more embarrassing. And it would prompt Mom to want to help me eat healthier. I appreciated her willingness to help, but I never had the willpower to stick to a diet for more than a few weeks at the most. Plus, the low-calorie food she ate looked gross. If eating that were the only way to slim down to a normal weight like my friends and other guys my age, then it would be impossible for me.

But moments like this deepened the horrible sense of self-disgust and self-hatred that tormented me beneath the facade of my life, which seemed so charmed in many other ways.

What made it worse was that I felt like what I'd been thinking all along—that the best thing I could possibly do was be just like my dad—was just plain wrong according to most of the world.

That night it was too hard to wrap my thirteen-year-old brain around these traumatic realizations. So when we went home, I played video games with Max. I also soothed my hurt feelings the best way I knew: with sweet treats like cookies. I'd eat them after our parents were asleep, so I wouldn't get any looks or comments from Mom about how I shouldn't be eating cookies after a big dinner or at night or at all. When she and Dad were sleeping, I'd enjoy as many chocolate chip cookies as I wanted, until the package was empty.

I loved the way the moist cookie sat on my tongue and began to dissolve while the chocolate chips oozed and my whole body reacted with an endorphin rush. I loved the feeling of my whole mouth being coated and full of the delicious chocolate flavor. Eating literally made me feel high. And that sweet distraction, while having fun with Max in the comfort of home, made the waitress and her comment feel a million miles away.

Focusing my energy on taste and secrecy and enjoyment

allowed me to put off until tomorrow, or another day, all the bad feelings and questions that I'd experienced in the restaurant.

I needed to avoid and deny what I'd only just begun to realize: the food that had always been synonymous with family love in my life was also the source of a whole lot of pain.

A SPECTACLE OF FOOD

Some of my best memories are of spectacular meals at my grandparents' ranch house. We went there every Thanksgiving, Christmas Eve, Christmas, and Easter.

Their finished basement was set up like a banquet hall—with its own kitchen!—to accommodate, as the family grew, forty or fifty aunts, uncles, and cousins. When we arrived, we always took off our shoes, and then went downstairs.

All the moms and aunts were cooking and setting up the buffet, while all the dads sat at long tables, talking, laughing, playing cards, or watching football. My grandmother's favorite Frank Sinatra music would be playing. Delicious scents of garlic and tomato filled the air.

Max and I hugged our grandparents, aunts, and uncles. Then we played cards or watched football with our twenty-seven cousins. We had no shame about eating everything, and more of everything. The buffet was better than any restaurant because everything was homemade with love. Ravioli, pizza, chicken, gravy and mashed potatoes, bread and butter, lasagna, sausage, meats, cakes, cannoli, and cookies.

Max and I would eat at least three plates of food. I ate fast, with no consciousness of how much food or how many calories I was consuming. I'd often feel bloated and nauseous afterward, yet I never thought, "Oh, I need to go on a diet." I just wanted my stomachache to go away.

At school I never felt teased or ostracized for being fat. I was popular—my schoolmates elected me class president in eighth grade. I saw myself as a successful student, like Dad was a successful businessman. I idolized everything about him and wanted to emulate him in every way—even his size. Max and I saw our dad as a big, strong man. I never saw him cry. I never saw him in pain. So I turned myself into that big, tough guy.

"We look just alike, Dad," I said proudly when I saw his first Communion picture, taken when he was in second grade. It thrilled me to hold my second-grade class picture beside it, because we looked like twins.

But by fifth grade, the embarrassment struck. Getting weighed in front of my classmates during gym class was, at the time, probably the most embarrassing moment I had ever experienced. A grown man can weigh two hundred pounds, not a ten-year-old boy. My cheeks would burn with shame, and I would just want to disappear as my friends stepped on the scale and registered normal weights.

At that point, I started to realize that being a huge man was not the ideal of strength, masculinity, and handsomeness I'd imagined it was. In gym class, I was slower and less agile. When we had to run the mile, I always came in last. The thin boys in my class ran it so fast and easily. Their stomachs were flat. Some had bony knees. I had a big belly, husky legs, and a full face. Why was I so different? Why couldn't I be like them?

Feeling bummed about being the fat kid made me want to eat—especially cookies. But cookies were making me fatter, which meant being even more embarrassed and disgusted with my big belly and thick thighs.

Around then, when I was ten, was when I became aware of the horrible cycle that trapped me in misery about my body. When I felt bad, I wanted to eat for comfort. This made me feel guilty and embarrassed that I was already fat and wanting cookies, so I'd eat secretly. I didn't want anyone to see me and snicker, "Look at that fat guy scarfing down cookies. Like he needs them!" Plus, I didn't want anyone or anything to interrupt my fascination with the textures, flavors, scents, visuals, and the endorphin rush of it all. Savoring food alone enabled me to focus on the enjoyment, without the self-consciousness or fear or scornful looks from people.

But the bingeing made me feel even worse, and the increasing size of my body meant that my secret eating was really no secret at all.

I was totally comfortable chowing down with my family; when I was with them I felt protected by a comfort zone where it was safe to eat huge portions. We took a lot of trips, which meant restaurants, buffets, and tons of car snacks. Either we were driving down to Atlanta to visit our grandparents; or going to the beach in North Carolina or Florida; or visiting museums in Washington, D.C.; or flying out to Las Vegas to escape the Michigan winter.

And since Dad was usually eating enormous portions, we did the same. We put buffets to shame. Technically, we ordered from the kids' menu, but we were eating more than man-size portions. At Chinese restaurant buffets, I devoured everything and anything fried, like almond chicken (it's battered, fried, and covered in sauce) and sweet and sour pork. At the Old Country Buffet, I feasted on everything but vegetables. I don't think I ate a salad until I was sixteen. Instead I wanted comfort foods like mashed potatoes and gravy, macaroni and cheese, fried chicken, fried fish, and desserts.

But when I was about twelve, and Max was ten, we decided that we wanted to lose weight.

"We can do it!" I whispered to Max. "We gotta go on a diet so we don't end up like him." Part of me felt like a traitor for not wanting to be like Dad anymore.

But I also felt an overwhelming need to protect Max from the pain I was experiencing. He had just told me that he'd had the same horrible experience of getting weighed in fifth grade.

"All the kids saw the scale go up to two hundred," Max said sadly. "I never want that to happen again."

"Next time I get weighed at school," Max said, "I want it to be around the same number as all the other boys."

"Let's start tomorrow," I said.

But we had no idea how to go on a diet. We only knew how to eat in a way that was making us fat. So we decided to talk with Mom. She was skinny, always eating salad and grilled chicken or fish, so we were sure she could help us.

"Mom, we want to lose weight," I cried. Max was crying too. "We need help."

She took us to a Weight Watchers program for kids, every Thursday after school. I was embarrassed and didn't tell any of my friends. I did okay, but I never exercised.

Max and I would stick with it for a while, but we still wanted to eat all the good stuff that we were used to. Plus Dad was always eating something good. So after a few days or weeks, we ditched the baked chicken and chowed down on pizza with Dad.

It caught up with me when I tried out for the basketball team in eighth grade. That required doing difficult exercises and running sprints to make sure I was fit enough to play. I didn't make the A-team. I made the B-team—the reject team. That season I had the most points, the most blocks, the most foul outs for the team. But we didn't win a single game. And being on the reject B-team really made me feel bad about myself.

At the end of eighth grade, I weighed 260. I hated the idea of starting high school and meeting girls, going to parties, or playing sports as the fat kid. And if I tried out for the basketball team, I wanted to make it.

So at my request, Mom took me back to Weight Watchers. First, though, we did what Mom and Dad always did when they started a diet. We took my "before" pictures, a full-length front view and side profile. I wore navy blue shorts, a yellow University of Michigan T-shirt, glasses, braces, and gym shoes. I was barrel shaped like my dad, with the fat concentrated in the middle.

Amazingly, I lost thirty pounds between eighth grade and high school. I made the cut for freshman football, and all those workouts really helped me drop some pounds.

Mom helped by shopping for healthy groceries and preparing low-calorie meals. Max hung with me for a while, but not for long. I could make it for spurts of two months at a time. Then I'd get bored and think, "You know what? I really want pizza." I'd eat it, and think, "I'll get back on my diet tomorrow." When tomorrow didn't come, I'd say, "I'll start at the end of the week." But then I would go to a birthday party and enjoy cake over the weekend. So I'd say, "Okay, Monday I'll get back on my plan." But I never did.

During my last semester in eighth grade, Dad had surgery to replace his hip. It tore me up inside to see him struggle. He never talked about it, but I could see that he was in pain. He went back to work for a while, but then he was home, with even more surgeries to clean out the split-open incision. As a thirteen-year-old kid who adores his dad, it was really tough to see him hooked up to an IV bag of antibiotics at home. I just wanted my dad to be well, but even then I was worried that his health would just get worse and worse and that we'd lose him too early.

I worried even more when I realized that I was just like him.

He was 350 pounds at age fifteen, and by the end of high school he was over 400.

I was starting high school, doomed to repeat the sins of my father.

I GAINED 150 POUNDS IN HIGH SCHOOL

When I turned sixteen, I got my driver's license. With a driver's license and a car—a burgundy Buick Century Custom that we inherited from my grandparents—I could go to any store or drive-through, whenever I wanted. And this became my formula for gaining 150 pounds—a whole person!—during high school.

Dad was busy with his new company and serving on the South Lyon City Council. Mom worked full time at the catering company. As a result, we rarely sat down to dinner together, unless we ate out.

Weekends in particular were calorie catastrophes.

On Friday nights, Max and I were free to eat whatever we wanted for dinner while Mom and Dad ate with friends at the South Lyon Hotel. After working at the pizzeria, I'd often come home with a giant meat lover's pizza and two tubs of chocolate chip cookie dough.

Max was my eating buddy. With him, there was no shame, no embarrassment, no worry. Our experiences with food and fat were so similar that eating together was simply our favorite sport.

We would devour the pizza in the family room while we watched TV. Then I'd dump an entire bucket of dough onto a cookie sheet and bake it into an enormous cookie. That one was for me. I'd make another one for Max. After we'd finished eating, I would hide the evidence under garbage in the bins outside our garage, where our parents would never notice. And they'd never know about the thousands of calories we had consumed while watching television and playing video games.

Max and I hid the evidence because we were old enough to know better. Even though we had buddies who could eat everything in sight, top it off with six desserts, and stay skinny as a rail, that was not our story. We ate a lot, and it showed. And even if our parents didn't harp on us to lose weight, there was still this weird dynamic: you tell your mom you want to lose weight, she takes you to Weight Watchers and buys you the healthy food, but then you give up and gain all the weight back, and then some.

Eating with wild abandon would announce to her and everyone else that we'd given up on trying to lose weight.

Embarrassment inspired our secrecy: it was too embarrassing to admit to anyone that the temptation of food's immediate gratification was far more powerful than our deep ache to lose weight.

It didn't help, either, that on Saturday and Sunday Max and I worked at McDonald's. I would eat the whole day's meals there. I'd usually grab the Deluxe Breakfast—pancakes, hash browns, scrambled eggs, sausage, and a biscuit. Then I'd make two breakfast burritos.

For lunch I'd have a twenty-piece box of Chicken McNuggets with all the sauces, like ranch and honey mustard. I'd also have a Double Cheeseburger and a McChicken, with fries and a Diet Coke. That lunch was probably 1,800 calories.

All day I worked in the food prep area, and I would literally pop chicken nuggets into my mouth during my entire shift. During breaks, I'd easily eat twenty-five chicken nuggets. Then, before my shift ended at 4:00 p.m., I'd grab two Double Cheeseburgers and a six-piece box of McNuggets. There was a gym just across the parking lot, in a strip mall, but I never made the connection that I should have been spending my time in the gym, working out, instead of in a fast-food restaurant, eating.

On school days, I'd skip breakfast so I could sleep later. For lunch I'd have whatever my mom packed, usually one or two turkey sandwiches, Jell-O, mandarin oranges, and pop. Then in the cafeteria I would also buy fries, and I'd eat whatever my friends didn't want.

Other than that, I ate the same size portions that other teenaged guys were eating.

In high school, my closet eating kicked into higher gear. I was fatter than everyone else, and I didn't want to give anyone the opportunity to pass judgment on me, criticize me, or be disgusted by me. Being so huge, it was embarrassing for people to see me eat. Our all-male school spared me the discomfort of eating in front of girls. After school I would retreat to the privacy of the car Max and I shared, and which left us free to stop at as many drive-throughs as we pleased.

He was my eating buddy, and our secrets were safe with each other. If he had something to do after school, I could eat alone, with my pick of Wendy's, McDonald's, or Taco Bell.

At home I'd do homework, then watch TV and play video games.

For dinner, if we weren't having pizza, going out, or having fast food, Mom cooked two dinners. For herself, she made chicken and steamed vegetables. For me, Max, and Dad, she made something like hamburgers. If only Max and I could have followed her excellent example of healthy eating, rather than stuff ourselves with garbage.

After dinner I'd make excuses to drive somewhere, so I could grab fifteen dollars worth of Wendy's or Taco Bell, which, when you think about the cost of fast food, was a huge amount of food.

I had accepted that this was me—a guy with a good life and a huge weight problem. I was going to eat, and I was going to eat a lot. It enabled me to numb myself to the guilt. I knew my body was being stretched and bulged in all the wrong directions. I hated that my belly was so big and that more and more fat was squeezing into the rolls on my back and into my double chin.

But I was so caught up in eating, and eating more to stuff down the bad feelings about being fat, that I just couldn't stop. I didn't want to stop. I just numbed myself to the negative and focused on the positive joy of eating.

I didn't get nauseous from eating so much. I never thought about the health problems that obesity would cause, even though I could look at Dad every day and see for myself. Maybe it sounds crazy or contradictory, but I was in such deep denial, and felt such teenaged invincibility, that I was able to function despite the torturous voices in my head saying, "I am so disgusted when I look at myself in the mirror. I hate how I struggle to move around. I have to lose weight, but I can't."

Then I'd think about the good things in my life and trick myself into thinking that everything was fine. I was getting straight As at school. I had a girlfriend from my sophomore year to my senior year. I had a close-knit group of guy friends who never made me feel different.

On a lot of levels, I had an awesome life.

I just accepted myself, thinking, "This is how I am. I'm still in high school. I can change eventually." But I had no idea when that would be.

During my senior year, I got accepted at Michigan State, which has a huge campus with about fifty thousand students and faculty members. It's located about an hour from home. I enrolled there and started preparing for my freshman year, when

I would start to study human biology with the aim of someday becoming a surgeon.

Just as I had dreaded the start of high school, I felt even worse about going to college.

I was literally wearing all those McNuggets, burgers, fries, pizzas, and chocolate chip cookies that I had sneaked when no one was looking. I may have been a closet eater, but more than ever the evidence of my secret binges was all over my body in a thick layer of fat. I knew that my weight would be the first thing people would see when I went to college, and I hated thinking about it.

I weighed 397 pounds at the end of my senior year.

I WANTED TO DIE

I was having a blast with my buddies at the all-night senior party in our school gymnasium. The music was booming and the 275 graduating seniors were shooting hoops, playing card games, and doing other fun things. Everybody was doing the Gladiator Joust, so I joined sixty guys who were standing around what looked like an inflatable blue boxing ring. We all cheered and shouted as our classmates whaled on each other with five-foot, Nerf-type foam batons. I was excited to get in there and battle.

Finally my turn came. I took one step into the ring, and the entire foam platform slowly descended into the inflatable base.

I wanted to die.

My heart was pounding. My face turned red. Nervous sweat prickled over my whole body.

I felt like I had turned into a four-hundred-pound freak show in front of the entire senior class.

All I could think was, "I have to change. I have to lose weight. I can't go to college like this."

My humiliation lasted two or three minutes, as I jousted with my classmate and the spectators made awkward jokes. Fortunately, since most of the guys were my friends and our school emphasized citizenship and kindness, nobody snickered. At least not that I could hear.

I just wanted to get through this stupid little gladiator fight, get off the mat, go hang out with my friends, and forget about it.

But I knew that wouldn't happen. The embarrassment of that moment would be forever burned into my mind and heart. I had to get real with myself. If I went to MSU in this fat suit, I would miss out on the great college experience of football games, pretty girls, and parties.

When I really thought about it, I had zero self-esteem and no sense of self-worth. When you're big, you give off a horrible first impression. People see your weight first. Why would any girls want to talk to me?

The problem was that I didn't see any way to change. Whenever I'd lost weight, with Mom's help, I gained it back. And losing thirty pounds was nothing compared to what I needed to drop now. It seemed like it would take me a million years to lose two hundred pounds—two hundred pounds!—by plain old diet and exercise.

How could I abandon a lifetime of eating enough for three or four people every day and stick to a regimen like Mom's?

Not to mention, I was planning to work at McDonald's all summer to save money for college. It would be impossible to work there and not scarf down chicken nuggets all day.

It would almost take divine intervention for me to change.

One morning, just a few weeks after the senior party, I was driving to work at three thirty in the morning to open the store.

"Do you have what it takes to become the biggest loser?" the radio announcer asked. I felt like he was talking directly to me. Dad had watched that show for years. "*The Biggest Loser* is holding auditions in metro Detroit . . ."

I turned up the volume to hear the details of where and when. This was divine intervention for me, Dad, and Max.

CHAPTER 7

MAX

Baseball Dreams Strike Out

We have a picture of me as a kid in which I look really happy because I'm enjoying two of my favorite things: eating and playing baseball. Wearing my Little League baseball uniform, I'm holding a gold trophy in one hand and a chocolate-covered ice cream bar in the other. I'm beaming with pride, with a giant grin. I still had my baby teeth, and there's some ice cream on my face.

I'm wearing a navy blue South Lyon Baseball T-shirt, and the whole picture has this totally all-American feeling. Behind me there's bright green grass, parents, and other kids. One mom is even wearing a red, white, and blue jacket.

I love that picture because I was so good at baseball that coaches from other teams would stop by my games or practices to watch me play. Oh, man, back when I was nine or ten, playing in Little League, it was the best. It was cool to be the big kid on the team—I was way stronger than all my friends, especially when we played T-ball. One time I was up to bat and all the coaches were rooting for me. I did like Babe Ruth—I pointed the bat to the outfield like that was where I was going to hit the ball.

I got a grand slam! The crowd and my family went wild! It was the coolest moment.

Then, like in so many pictures of me in my baseball uniform, I had this look in my eyes while I was holding a bat, like it was only a matter of time before the American League would be mine. Plus, I loved that my mom, dad, and brother were always there to cheer me on.

But there's something else you'd notice if you looked at that picture of me with the trophy and ice cream bar.

I'm chubby. I already have a double chin, and my belly is pressing over the waistband of my jeans.

If a picture speaks a thousand words, then this one says, "Max Morelli is on his way to obesity, not the big leagues."

And it's true: by the time I hit adolescence, weighing well over two hundred pounds, I was too fat to play baseball. Every time I ran, I'd get out of breath and feel like it was impossible to move fast. So I quit.

I was really bummed, but not bummed enough to stop eating. I'd lost one of my favorite pursuits, but I sure wasn't going to give up the other. Food, lots of food, was a huge part of life in the Morelli family. As a kid I loved to chow on pizza, burgers, and fries, as all kids do. Just like my brother, I wanted to be like our dad and the big men in our family. But by the time I realized that too big was not better, the damage was done. My brain and body were already programmed to consume massive amounts of food and to carry those extra calories around as thick layers of fat.

I was like a younger carbon copy of my brother when it came to eating and food. The only difference was that Michael was shy about eating in front of people outside of the family. Me? I'd pull a chair up to a buffet and dig in if I could. I didn't care. I just wanted to eat as much as possible, and it didn't matter who saw me.

Fortunately, it seemed like life was always offering up one more chance to chow down in a big way: meals at home and at restaurants with my family, holidays at my grandparents' house, and family vacations. As a kid growing up, I was having too much fun and feeling too much love to feel like anything was wrong with our lifestyle.

Even when we stopped eating at the kitchen table, when I was around eight, in third grade, I thought it was cool. What kid wouldn't rather eat in front of the TV in the family room? Our family life was moving at a hectic pace. Mom was working full time. Dad was working a lot, with meetings on some nights. Michael had Cub Scouts. We both had baseball, soccer, and basketball.

So all of a sudden, instead of Mom cooking we would just grab McDonald's, or Dad would bring home a pizza, or we'd go to the South Lyon Hotel or the Mexican place in town.

And I just kept getting bigger. I was becoming just like my dad and uncles, and just like my brother. I thought that was awesome for most of my younger years. A lot of our experiences and feelings were identical. The major differences between us were that my brother was a lot more of an inside person. He'd rather play video games like Pokémon or card games inside the house. As for me, I'd rather be outside playing Frisbee. Another difference is that Michael has a huge sweet tooth; I don't at all. I'd rather eat real food, like burgers and pizza.

It was a joke in our family that ketchup was my favorite vegetable. Dad even used to buy me giant bottles of ketchup as gag gifts. If I ever ate a salad in a restaurant, I'd order extra ranch dressing and drown the lettuce in 600 calories worth of fat.

Like most kids, we had no concept of calories. We just knew what tasted good and what didn't. I had a carefree attitude about it until I was ten. That's when it really hit me that I was fat.

"I weigh two hundred pounds!" I cried when Mom picked me up from school. "I can't believe I'm in fifth grade and I weigh two hundred pounds!" That was my worst experience in elementary school, because I had to get weighed in gym class, in front of all the other kids.

Seeing that I was more than double the weight of my buddies was just horrible. That's probably the moment when I started hating my weight. I hated that it weighed me down and stopped me from being a great baseball player. I hated that it made me gasp for air and sweat bullets during gym class, when games like kickball or flag football seemed easy for my friends. I hated the thick, fleshy feeling of my arms and legs. I would look at my skinny friends and wonder why I couldn't down pizza, burgers, and ice cream and stay skinny like they did. I hated that I was such a fun-loving guy trapped in a huge body that slowed me down.

But I saw no way to change.

So I kept eating.

TOO FAT TO RIDE

Ever since I was little, I'd been going to Cedar Point Amusement Park with my family. Every year, as I got older, I could go on bigger and better rides. The bumper cars, the Tilt-a-Whirl, the Blue Streak, the Demon Drop. This place had the best roller coasters, and I was so excited to get big enough to ride them. So when I got to go there for a school trip to celebrate the end of eighth grade, I was thrilled. Going on all those rides with my buddies would be a blast!

Little did I know, I had actually gotten too big.

The Corkscrew was the coolest ride in the park: it looped in corkscrews over people walking on the sidewalks. You'd be fly-ing up the sides, then upside down, then flying up into the next loop. I remembered how fun it was on previous trips.

"Dude, this is the best!" my friend said, as we each lowered a padded metal harness over our heads and shoulders. It was like an upside-down U that clamped down and locked over your chest to hold you in during the upside-down parts of the ride.

"Yeah!" I answered my friend, as I pulled down the harness. But it wouldn't go down over my belly, so it wouldn't lock.

"I'm sorry," the attendant said. "You can't ride."

My face felt hot with embarrassment. My buddies, and the huge line of people, were witnessing the most humiliating moment of my thirteen-year-old life: I was too fat to ride.

I wished I could disappear. It felt like I was moving in slow motion as I raised the harness and stood up. I was sure that some jerk in line would make a "fat boy" comment. And I knew all those cute girls would have either disgust or pity in their eyes, so I didn't dare look over there.

"Sorry, dude," said my buddy in the next seat.

"It's okay," I said, stepping onto the platform. "See ya at the end."

But it wasn't okay. I wanted to cry or let the attendant know I was pissed off that the ride wasn't big enough for me. But I couldn't cry or show that I was pissed off, because everybody was watching and nobody wants to be the crybaby with a temper tantrum when you're hanging out with your friends.

My mind was spinning in a thousand bad directions as I stepped off the platform. The end of eighth grade means you're almost done with middle school. Then you head off to high school, where you transform from a kid to a man. Would I just keep getting big-ger and end up like my dad?

I could hear my friends hollering with excitement as the ride whooshed them away for a few minutes of fun. I walked over to the exit gate and waited for them to finish.

"This sucks," I told myself. "I gotta lose weight."

But I felt so hopeless. And furious. I was too fat to fit a ride that easily held adult men. Tears blurred my vision; I quickly rubbed them away.

"Hey, dude, let's get some chow," my buddy said as they got off the ride.

Minutes later the pain and embarrassment, and the desperate wish to lose weight, disappeared from my thoughts because the burger, fries, and Sprite I bought tasted so good. I didn't think about anything except whether I'd go back for seconds.

Fortunately, I'd been friends with the same guys since kindergarten, so they never made fun of me. They accepted me as Max. But they could do so many more things than I could—play sports and run fast.

Another difference? Girls. When you're thirteen, you like girls. And you want them to like you back.

"Oh, Max, you're such a good friend," they would always say. They could never see me as anything more than a friend. But they would flirt all day long with my buddies.

I also didn't dress as cool as the other boys. They shopped at normal stores like Target and Walmart. But I had to shop with my dad and brother at the "big and tall" men's store. At school, we wore a uniform—khaki pants and white shirts. The only difference with me was that my uniform was much bigger. Just because we wore the same clothes didn't mean I blended in, though. It's impossible to blend in with the rest of the guys when you're double their size.

I was depressed sometimes, thinking, "I can't do this." Or "Girls don't like me." I felt angry at myself for getting this way,

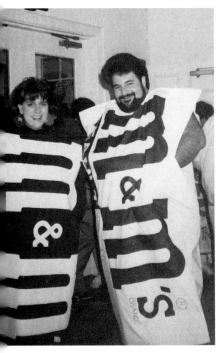

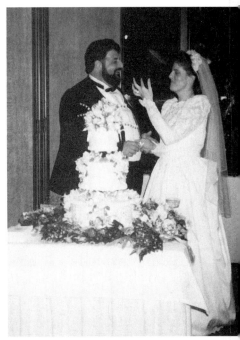

Becky and Ron at Structure House's Halloween party. We spent hours making these costumes.

October 8, 1988. Our wedding reception. We had crept back into our old eating habits and were gaining weight slowly but surely.

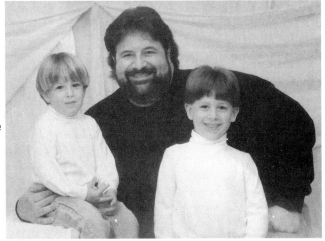

Ron surprised Becky for her birthday by taking the boys to get this portrait made. Ron's knee hurt for weeks afterward.

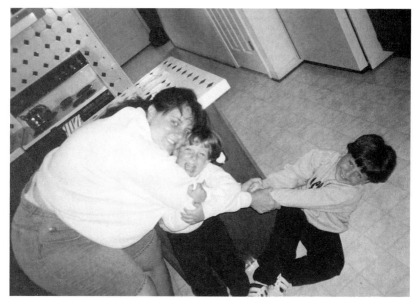

Becky and the boys being silly. We had decided that we would never make a big deal about the boys' eating habits or weight. We were naive to think that they wouldn't mimic our penchant for huge portions or fattening foods.

Max's fourth birthday—the ultimate boy's fantasy cake made with chocolate "dirt" and trucks!

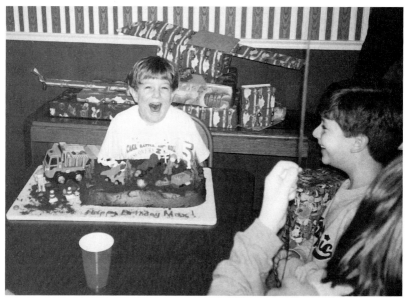

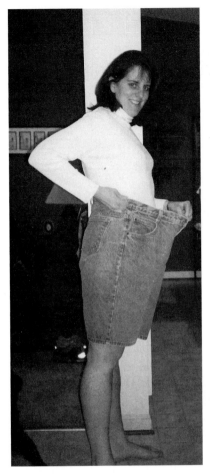

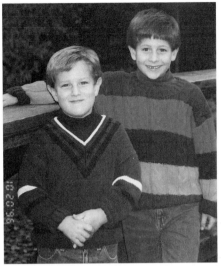

This photo was used for our Christmas card in 1996. Michael was six years old and Max was four.

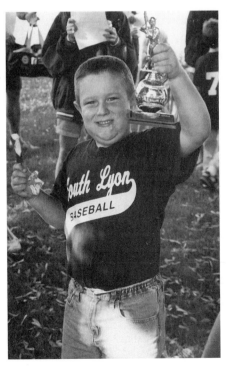

Each time a family member attempted to lose weight, we would stand in front of this column in the kitchen. This photo was taken in July 1997, after Becky's bariatric surgery.

Max at age nine, during his Little League glory days, enjoying two of his favorite things: ice cream and baseball.

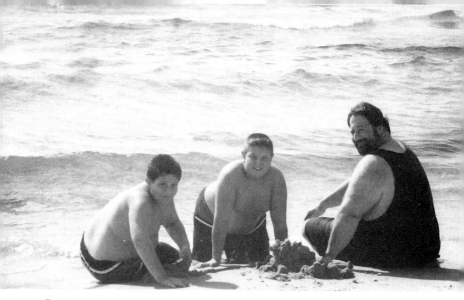

Ron and the boys playing in the sand in Ludington, Michigan, during a beach trip up north. The boys were eleven and nine years old.

Our vacation at Universal Studios. The scooter made it much easier for us to tour the park, but it was sad that Ron had come to that.

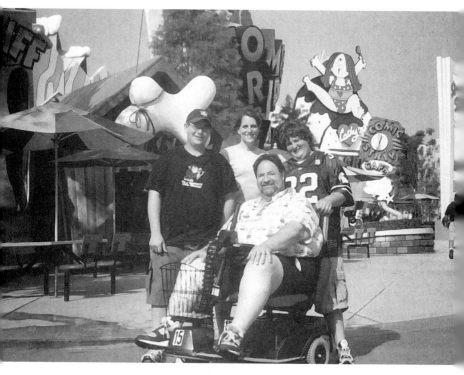

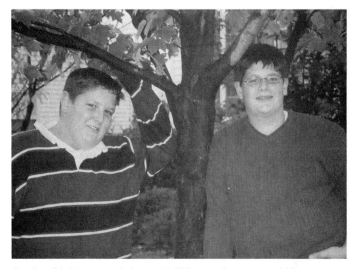

Another Christmas card shot, with Mike age fourteen and Max age twelve.

The boys leaving for Mike's high school graduation. Bob Harper later saw this picture of Max and thought it was so sad, because he looks like a middle-aged man instead of the young teen that he was.

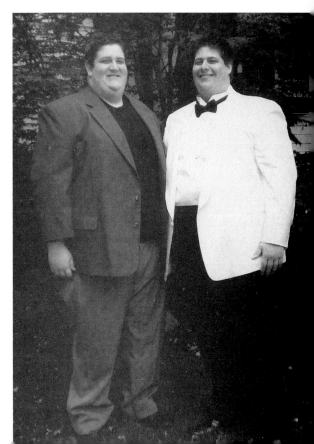

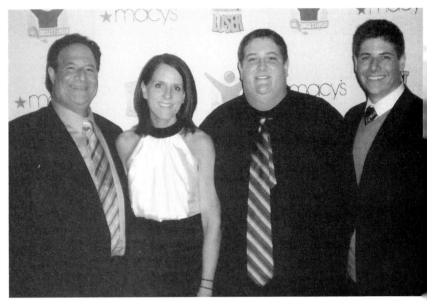

The family after the "reveal" on the makeover show. Millions of people watched as Max broke down, telling Michael how sad he was to be the only "big" one left in the family.

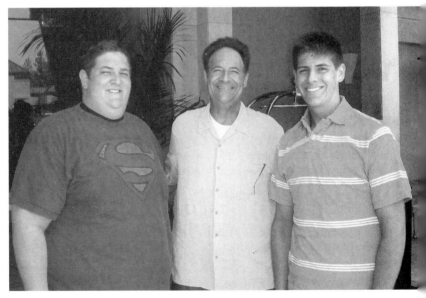

Ron and the boys leaving the hotel after getting their spray tans for the show's finale. Who would have ever thought? It's so LA!

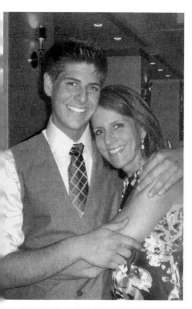

Becky gives Michael a big hug at the party after the finale.

Max on our family cruise in August 2010. He looks great after losing another seventy pounds at Fitness Ridge.

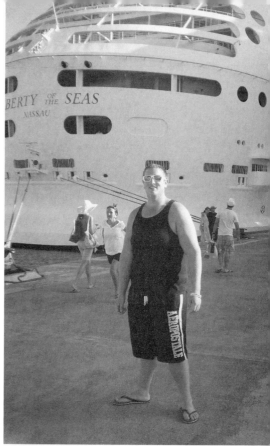

Bob Harper and Mike at the *Biggest Loser* finale party. Bob was a huge source of inspiration for both Mike and Ron throughout the show.

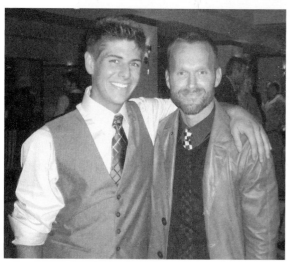

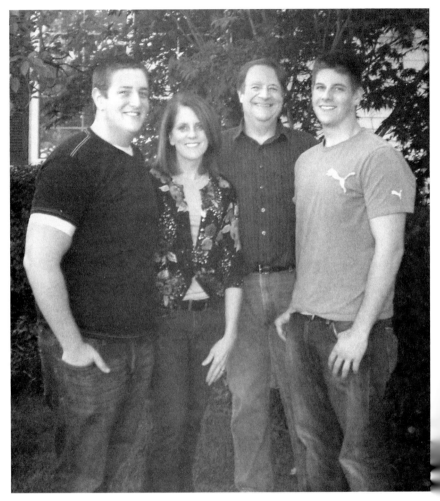

The family looking and feeling great on Ron and Becky's twenty-second wedding anniversary in October 2010.

but instead of dealing with it I kept eating, and it got worse and worse.

IT WAS JUST NORMAL TO EAT A LOT

Of course Michael and I tried to diet, but it was too hard. I'd been eating the good stuff for as long as I could remember. For a kid whose favorite vegetable was ketchup, salads and baked chicken just didn't satisfy my hunger. It was too hard for me to learn delayed gratification because I'd always had immediate gratification. We had no rules to get in the way of snacks and meals.

Maybe it sounds weird that we didn't know how to lose weight, since our parents were always either gaining or losing. But I was only three when Dad had gastric bypass surgery and four when Mom had it. So I don't remember them going through that.

I do remember vacations where we were all eating whatever we wanted. Then all of a sudden Mom was a health food fanatic. Her food looked gross. Dad's food looked great. We never stopped and said, "Okay, we have to do something about this. Now. Together."

So Michael and I just carried on, sometimes having our tearful secret meetings, but for the most part we continued to eat like it was an Olympic sport.

THE HIGH SCHOOL YEARS: FUN BUT FATTENING

At the end of my sophomore year in high school, I weighed almost four hundred pounds. So did Michael, who was a senior about to graduate.

Even though I hated being fat, I still had a lot of fun in school. I was known as a jokester, and I had tons of friends who accepted me just the way I was.

At our homecoming assembly during my sophomore year, we had a tug-of-war competition. I told my whole class that if we beat the junior class, I'd do the Soulja Boy dance in front of the whole school.

During the tug-of-war, the entire tenth grade was in the bleachers chanting, "Max! Max! Max!"

We beat the juniors, and I danced across the gym floor, doing this really cool hip-hop dance that has a sort of Superman dive at the end. It was wild. It was crazy. It was me. I was always up to some crazy antics that had people laughing.

Like when I painted my face blue and cheered louder than anyone in the gym during the basketball game. Sometimes my mischief got me in a little trouble: one casual-dress day, for instance, I wore black spandex from head to toe. The teachers were not too happy about that—I got sent home to change into normal clothes. But I was tamer when playing in the student-faculty basketball game and acting in a skit for the seniors.

I loved feeling that other kids liked me because I was fun, no matter what I looked like. But if you think about the phrase "the tears of a clown," that kind of described me. Just below my seemingly happy surface, I hated being obese. If, alone in my room, I sat still long enough to think about it, I would get depressed. I was terrified to think that I would never lose weight. That I'd grow up and be as huge as Dad, and never have a girlfriend or go on dates or do the fun romantic stuff that guys were supposed to do.

Just like my brother, it was easier for me to stop thinking about all the bad stuff by eating. It was really the best remedy. I'd go down from my room to the kitchen, get a bag of chips and dip, and eat. Or I'd hit a drive-through for a bag of burgers and fries. It's like my brain had an automatic response, like when you e-mail somebody and immediately get a message back saying they're away on vacation.

For my brain it was like: Bad thought? Eat.

Then while I was eating, if the bad thought tried to return, I'd think about what I'd eat when I'd finished with the chips or burgers. Then I'd get so full it would mellow me out, and it would be easier to just lie on the couch and watch TV or play a video game. Then the next day would come, and I'd feel bad that I kept eating, and those bad feelings would make me eat even more. Making it even worse was the fact that I was doing it to myself. Nobody was making me eat that much, but I felt like my brain and body were programmed to be that way. I wished I knew of a way to deprogram my head, but that seemed impossible.

Making matters worse, the typical school day brought with it a lot of reminders that I was morbidly obese.

Whenever I needed to use my student ID, I got a quick reminder of how much weight I'd gained since the picture was taken, only a few months before. From year to year, my face got fatter and fatter, and I could see it if I compared the pictures on the annual IDs. It was ridiculous. I first noticed it between freshman and sophomore year, when I was fifteen and working at McDonald's.

So on many nights, I would eat there while working, and then stop at Taco Bell on the way home. I'd go to bed with all that grease and salt in my stomach. The next morning, I'd skip breakfast and wish I weighed half what I did. It was like this constant fantasy was playing in my head, while my actions continued to reinforce the reality that I hated.

Then I'd hurry to class in the crowded hallway. If anyone ever said something about my weight, I'd get really pissed. Like once when I bumped into a guy by accident.

"Hey, watch it!" the kid snapped.

"Watch where you're goin'!" I said.

"Maybe if you weren't so *fat*—"

I turned around and got in his face. The bulk of my body intimidated him because he stepped back, looking scared, toward the locker.

"Hey, dude, no biggie," he said, his hands up. "It's cool."

"Keep it that way," I ordered before storming away.

My hair-trigger temper could get set off so easily, especially if someone said something about my weight. I already hated the way I looked and felt, and I definitely didn't need some other guy to point it out to me. When you're fat, it's like you wear the problem for all the world to see, yet you want to deny just how bad it is.

And I could see that all the things that TV, the movies, and magazines held up as attractive about a teenage guy were the opposite of me. Attractive guys were slim and buff. I was huge. And that made me feel ugly.

So every day, all these thoughts and feelings exploded inside my head. And when a kid said something to me about it, all that anger came bursting out.

I fumed all the way to the cafeteria. I was able to chill out a little bit when I saw my friends at lunch, though. I sat down at our usual table and ate two peanut butter sandwiches and chips, then went into the cafeteria line and bought pizza and fries.

"Hey, Max, you had me rollin' the other night," my buddy said. "You're a regular comedian."

I smiled, remembering what a good time we'd all had at our friend's house, just hangin' out, talking and watching TV. Lunch with my friends was always fun—it helped me forget about stuff like the kid in the hallway.

But then it was back to class and squeezing into one of those all-in-one chair-desk torture devices; it was enough to enrage me again.

It was so weird how my moods could change from one minute to the next. At home my mother or brother would say something to infuriate me, but then I'd play a video game and mellow out just as fast.

Like one night, Dad was getting on me about college. I snapped and shouted, "You can't tell me to go to college if you didn't go to college!"

Another time he told me I shouldn't eat tortilla chips and cheese dip when I wanted a snack after school.

"You can't tell me what to eat!" I yelled, as if he had flipped a mad switch on for me. I had no control over my moods.

Or eating. A lot of my eating happened in the car. I was always on my way to get something to eat, eating it, driving to meet my friends to eat, or coming home with food. Weight gain was making it uncomfortable to drive because it was hard to get in and out of the car and the steering wheel was pressing into my belly, but that didn't stop me from the drive-through binges.

If my friends and I got hungry, we'd go to McDonald's at midnight. I'd have three Double Cheeseburgers and two McChickens. My calorie count just for that meal would be around 2,500 or 3,000.

At other times, after school, I'd hang out with my friends at Wendy's, where I would eat two bacon double cheeseburgers and two ninety-nine-cent chicken sandwiches. If we went to Taco Bell, I ate a Crunchwrap Supreme. My buddies and I would also go to Buffalo Wild Wings, where I would eat sixteen boneless wings and fries.

I always felt sick afterward, but I didn't really care enough to change the way I ate. I felt hopeless. And reckless. For a while, I made myself throw up after every meal so I didn't gain weight. I'd heard about girls doing it so they could eat fattening stuff and not gain weight. So I tried it. The whole time, I had this bad feeling like I was doing something I really shouldn't have been doing. But even that didn't help.

In fact, my best friend called me out because he was worried. He kept tabs on his phone of how many times I threw up. He said, "That's seven times in two weeks, when I've been around." I stopped after he said that. I felt like I was going from bad to worse, and it wasn't even helping me lose weight.

Food was making me lose out on even more fun, though. I got too fat to play sports. I'd stopped playing baseball and basketball; instead I played football during my freshman year. I loved it, but I hurt my back, then didn't play sophomore year. I was going to play junior year, but I dislocated my knee and then tore two tendons in it. After that I was manager of the basketball team.

At home after school, it was easy to hide what we ate because Mom was at work. For a while, Dad was at home, after he sold his business. But he never stopped us from eating whatever we wanted, because he was eating pizza, peanut butter, and fast food too.

Deep down, I felt horrible about my weight. But I didn't see any way to change it. I'd tried diets, and I just couldn't stick to them. So I just kept eating.

CHAPTER 8

/ **MIKE AND RON**

The Chance of a Lifetime

Mike
Despite the Rain, We Shined for the Judges

I was so embarrassed about our plans to audition for *The Biggest Loser* that I didn't tell my girlfriend, my friends, or my boss at McDonald's. Somehow the obvious fact that I was morbidly obese, and that I desperately wanted to lose weight, was just too overwhelming to talk about. The very thought roused all that horrible embarrassment that was always gnawing at me.

But after hearing the ad for the auditions, which were just twenty minutes from our house, it seemed like the only escape route from my four-hundred-pound fat suit before I hit the college scene.

I thought, "We have to go to the audition, get picked, lose the weight, and win!" The $250,000 prize would be nice, but the real motivator was the priceless thrill of finding the thin, young, muscular guy that I'd never seen in my mirror.

"Hey," I said to my boss the next day at work, where I was on the early-morning shift, preparing to open the restaurant for breakfast. "Dad wants to surprise me tomorrow. Can I get off early, at 8:00 a.m.?" My boss said yes!

I was so excited as we drove to the Gardner-White Furniture Store, in nearby Canton, for the audition.

"Oh no!" I said as I drove through the parking lot toward a line of about two hundred people that wrapped around the building. Then it started to rain. Hard. In the car, Dad and I watched in disbelief and silence. Then we looked at each other.

"Do we really want to do this?" Dad asked.

"We're already here," I said. "Why give up?" But then I thought about how uncomfortable it would be for him to stand in line, because his knees hurt all the time.

"Dad, we don't have to do this if you don't want to. We can apply online."

My dad looked at me like he would never let me down. He could obviously see that I wanted to do this more than anything I had ever wanted in my life.

RON
We Had to Try

All that hope and desperation in my son's eyes made me think, "I'm going to do this for my son." Still, I never thought we'd make the show.

"Let's do it," I said. We hadn't eaten breakfast, so we went to the nearby White Castle. Then we braved the line—and the rain—for six hours. Despite our umbrella, we got soaked. It was interesting to see the people; after watching the primetime TV show, I had an idea of what former contestants looked like—wholesome, clean-cut, well-spoken, and appealing to mainstream viewers. Here at the audition, most of the people lacked that look. But this observation didn't exactly overwhelm me with confidence that we'd get picked.

Standing there gave me a lot of time to think.

"I'm eating myself to death."

That thought had rung like a death knell in my head when I should have been enjoying one of my proudest moments: Michael's high school graduation.

We had joined hundreds of people in Hill Auditorium in Ann Arbor. Amid the priests in black suits and collars and the graduates in white tuxedos, Michael strode across the stage to receive his diploma. Tears of pride filled my eyes, but guilt and fear came crushing down on me as I squeezed into the chair alongside Max and Becky.

At 430 pounds, my physical discomfort was a constant reminder of my failure. As a father. As a husband. And as the person I had to live with inside this enormous body.

That day was a huge wake-up call. It was a sunny spring morning in May, exactly twenty-one years after Becky and I had met at Structure House. Before coming to commencement, we had taken pictures of Michael and Max at home, on our front lawn. Looking at them, I thought, "My God, look what I did to my kids."

I felt horrible. I had just turned fifty-four, and my body was giving out. Would I live to see Michael graduate from Michigan State? What about medical school? Would I survive two more years to see Max graduate from high school? What about their weddings? Would excess food and fat kill me before I became a grandfather?

As I watched Michael with his buddies at graduation, I wondered how long it would be before he and Max were popping pills, taking shots, and sleeping in masks.

Still on the South Lyon City Council, I was also doing consulting work and driving a bus for our city's school district. I absolutely loved working with the kids.

But now every time I looked at my own kids I was ashamed of being a foodaholic father.

I felt worse when I looked at slim, fit Becky. I had been tormenting her all these years by enabling the boys to eat with me. If only we all could have followed her excellent lead as a healthy role model. Rather than commend her, though, I resented her. Becky's discipline had taken the fun out of our relationship.

"This isn't the person I married," I often thought. We were just tolerating each other. I stopped saying "I love you" and we lost the desire for affection.

So there we were. A fat family with a skinny mom. We were all miserable.

Now Michael and I stood in the pouring rain for a shot at the one-in-a-million opportunity to be on *The Biggest Loser*. The show seemed like our only hope.

"Hey, guys, how's it goin' today?" asked Pete Thomas, the "at-home" winner of $100,000 during the show's second season. Contestants who are eliminated from the show still have a chance to become the "at-home" winner by continuing to lose weight at home, then getting weighed at the finale. The previously eliminated contestant who has lost the largest percentage of body weight becomes the "at-home" winner.

Meeting someone who had done that made me stare in awe. Pete was fit and radiantly healthy. He was everything Michael and I dreamed of being. And *The Biggest Loser* had gotten him there. Excitement jolted through me.

"When you get inside," he told us, "you'll see the judges and you'll fill out some papers, okay?"

I was a little starstruck. Watching him on our TV in the family room, and witnessing his dramatic 185-pound weight loss, made me admire him even more.

"I remember *you*," I said as we shook Pete's hand.

Then Pete said, "Hey, wait, are you a father-and-son team?"

"Yeah, I'm Ron."

"I'm Mike. We're from South Lyon. I'm eighteen."

"Cool, cool," Pete said.

Mike
I Wanted It So Bad!

The way Pete looked at us made me think, "Oh my God! We're gonna make the show."

I just knew it, right then. But we still had to formally face the judges inside the furniture store. When we finally reached the back area, two casting people were sitting on one side of a pair of big tables, evaluating about ten potential contestants at once. They asked our name, age, and weight. We also had to fill out a questionnaire.

"I want to be a surgeon," I told the judges. They asked about me going to college and why I wanted to be a surgeon. The attention we got felt like an eternity compared to the nanoseconds they spent with everyone else.

"Wait, *how* old are you?" a casting person asked me.

"I'm eighteen," I said confidently. I knew my age made me stand out from the other people.

"I feel good about that," Dad said as we walked to the car. "We did pretty well. If we get a callback in the next three days, it'll be okay."

He was wrong. As soon as I turned on my cell phone in the car, it rang.

"Can you guys come to another casting call at the Embassy Suites Hotel in two days?" Pete Thomas asked.

I knew it!

Two days later, Dad and I upgraded from the casual clothes we had worn to the audition; now we sported dress shirts and jackets for on-camera interviews with the casting people.

"This should take thirty to forty-five minutes," they said.

They interviewed us for ninety minutes.

"I can't go on living like this," I said on camera. "I can't be four hundred pounds and eighteen years old. I can't be a surgeon and be four hundred pounds, because my stomach wouldn't let me reach the operating table." Hearing myself tell my tragic tale of fat and food made me cry. Dad too. It was very intense.

And in my gut, I just *knew*.

BECKY
The Summer of Hurry Up and Wait

We were having a barbecue to celebrate my birthday on July 2, and our house was full of friends who were thrilled that Ron and Michael were being considered for *The Biggest Loser*.

I was really excited, but cautious because I didn't want us to get our hopes up.

The producers had asked for video of Ron and Michael interacting with their family and friends. We didn't own a camcorder, and they wanted us to send the video to California ASAP. So we borrowed a camera and tapped a friend's editing skills. The party was over, and we were videotaping scenes of Michael and Ron doing this and that around the house. They started arguing about a computer function, and I was tempted to turn off the camera. But I kept it on. They were auditioning for a "reality" show, after all, and this was a real-life father-and-son situation.

"You're an idiot!" Ron shouted on camera.

"No, you're an idiot!" Mike yelled back.

We sent in the video and didn't hear anything for weeks. At that point, we thought, "It's over. We're out. No chance."

"They're not gonna pick you," I told Ron, who had just been diagnosed with a torn rotator cuff. "You could never do all those challenges on the show. You're so sick and on all this medication."

I was also afraid that his gastric bypass surgery would get him disqualified, because we thought it wasn't allowed. But Ron had characterized it as yet another weight-loss failure.

We had almost given up hope when a producer called, asking for Ron and Michael to get a physical right away. They did it, sent in the paperwork, and again we heard nothing for weeks. Would they get picked? Or not?

Talk about high anxiety!

Meanwhile, we were getting ready for the biggest transition of Michael's life: his first year of college. We were shopping for things for the dorm room, packing, planning, and all the while not knowing whether he'd actually go to college or be chosen for *The Biggest Loser*.

September came. Michael went to East Lansing. And we still didn't know if he and Ron were going to be on the show.

Mike
I Was Ecstatic

I was still so embarrassed that I didn't tell my college-dorm suite-mates that I'd auditioned for *The Biggest Loser*. As thrilled as I was to be at college, I hated that I was embarking on this new part of my life as an obese guy. That's all people could see as I walked across campus to my classes or met new people in my dorm. My self-consciousness and lack of self-esteem totally overshadowed the fun. Eating in the dorm was so uncomfortable; I felt like everybody was looking at what the fat guy was putting on his tray. Being a closet eater is impossible with roommates because you're rarely alone. So I wasn't even able to indulge my favorite habit of secretly eating cookies to feel better for a moment.

All the while, I kept hoping that *The Biggest Loser* would call after all, and that Dad and I would be chosen for the show. We hadn't heard anything. Not getting chosen would plunge me into a really bad mental place, and I feared I would just give up on ever becoming thin and happier and trying to enjoy college life to the fullest.

Amazingly, eight days into the semester, on September 7, 2008, a casting guy called while we were playing the video game NCAA Basketball 2009. I went into another room to talk in private.

"Pack for five months, Mike," he said, "because you're coming to California!"

"Yeah!" I shouted. I felt like I would explode with excitement. The catch? Dad and I would have to participate in a final audition; we could get sent home after a week or two. In my mind, though, I knew we'd make it. All the way.

I called Dad's cell phone. Busy. I called home.

"You guys are going to California!" Max cheered. It meant so much to me that my brother was excited for me. I didn't want him to feel jealous or left out. And I felt guilty about his weight because of all those times that I'd supplied the pizza and cookie dough for our Friday night binges. Hopefully, if we could stay on long enough to succeed, then our success would inspire his too.

I returned to my suitemates and said, "This is my last game of NCAA. I'm going to California!"

My friends looked excited but confused.

"Have you guys heard of the show *The Biggest Loser*?" I asked. Their faces lit up and they nodded and said, "Yeah."

"I might be on it!" I exclaimed. So much hope and excitement was exploding in me that my embarrassment melted away. This let everybody know that I truly wanted to lose weight, and that it was now a huge possibility.

All four of them whooped and cheered.

"Dude, you'd be perfect for that show!" one shouted.

I loved hearing encouragement from my new friends. Suddenly, I wasn't embarrassed to tell my boss and people at work. They were super supportive. It was great knowing that people wanted me to succeed because they cared about me and my well-being.

I was ecstatic! I felt like I had a real shot now. I kept thinking, "Here's where I'm gonna lose all my weight, get healthy, and change my life."

Everyone who is overweight thinks that if they were fit, their life would be as perfect as in the movies. I always thought about the college scenes in *American Pie* and ached down to my bones to experience something like that. The superhot girls, the fun parties, the good times. Now if I were chosen for the show, I hoped to get my chance to find out if fit guys really did have more fun in college.

I told my professors that I was leaving. Then Dad came to campus, and we dealt with the registrar. That's when it really hit me that I was in limbo. Despite my confidence, it was a big gamble to leave my freshman year of college for a *maybe*, albeit the best *maybe* of my life.

RON
California Dreamin'

Five days later, Michael and I were on an airplane. We insisted that *The Biggest Loser*'s travel coordinators buy us three seats, so that we could have an empty seat between us. They were sending eight hundred pounds of flesh to California, which would not fit in two seats. I knew to make this request because Becky and I had done the same thing when she was big and we'd take airplane trips together.

Next came the more humiliating request: "We need two seat-belt extenders," I told the flight attendant. My heart pounded with embarrassment because other passengers could hear me.

Michael—wearing size 56 jeans—was silent.

But judging by the determination in his eyes as we ascended, I knew we'd be gone a long time. We'd even applied for absentee ballots for the upcoming presidential election between Democratic senator Barack Obama and Republican senator John McCain. We were optimistic that we would not be home on November 4— more than a month away—to vote.

"We'll never have to use these again," I told Michael as we attached the seat-belt extenders and fastened them over our huge bellies.

"Never," Michael agreed. "Dad, let's set a goal to lose three hundred pounds between us."

"Deal," I said. "I think we're going to come home as half the men we are now."

Michael grinned. "I'm ready to make that happen! We'll never fall below the yellow line. And we're going all the way to the finale. I just *know* it."

I loved Michael's confidence. But I never thought I could make it through the challenges or intense workouts for six months.

I was sick and broken, but I was ready to help my son become the Biggest Loser.

Max
So Excited, So Worried

Suddenly Mom and I were home alone, and we were so excited that Dad and Michael were going on national TV.

I felt nervous for them, though. One minute I'd be like, "They'll make it to the end of the show and lose all their extra weight." But then I'd remember Dad's health problems and think, "I hope they don't get sent home in a week." I felt like my success depended on theirs.

My mom was so cool about it, saying that I would be the man of the house while they were gone. Plus, I'd get the car to drive to school and work.

"This is a great time to focus on being healthy and making changes here at home," Mom said. "We can both eat better and exercise while they're gone." We went to the grocery store and stocked up on healthy foods. I thought that was a great idea. I had this picture in my head of going to the gym, eating like Mom, and being a much thinner guy when they returned thin too. I would be proud of them, they would be proud of me, and it would be awesome.

Mike
We're Going to the Ranch!

It was amazing that Dad and I made it to the top 100 people out of the 250,000 who had auditioned all across America. Now we were quarantined in the Sheraton Universal Hotel in Los Angeles, where we did interviews and on-camera screen tests. It felt like producers and casting staff were evaluating whether we were genuine and if our story would create good reality TV.

I felt confident and comfortable that Dad and I would be among the twenty-two lucky people who'd get chosen for the show. In fact, I ended up talking with the senior story producer and didn't even know it. He was wearing a Red Sox hat, and I told him how much I liked the Red Sox. I had no idea that months later he would actually give me that very hat.

One day we were with twenty other people doing an on-camera screen test when *The Biggest Loser*'s host, Alison Sweeney, entered the room looking serious.

"You've come a long way," she said, "and I'm sorry to tell you, you're going to have to pack your bags and leave this hotel . . . because you're all going to the ranch!"

Yes! I knew it! Dad and I hugged. Everyone around us was jumping up and down, hugging, screaming.

"You made it!" Alison said. "You're going to the ranch. Here's your chance to change your life."

For both of us, this was probably the happiest time of the entire experience. Our emotions were like an explosion of excitement, shock, optimism, and gratitude. We felt energized with pure euphoria that we were getting a priceless opportunity to shrink our bodies, reprogram our brains, and leave our fat, food-addicted lives behind forever.

As a symbol of that transition, we changed into black shorts and milk-chocolate-colored T-shirts with *The Biggest Loser* logo. It was official; we were now the Brown Team, and we couldn't wait to get to work.

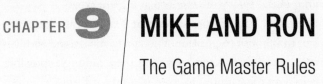

MIKE AND RON
The Game Master Rules

RON
I Was Controlling Relationships to Help Michael

The Godfather.

Ron the Don.

The Hatchet Man.

I never imagined that our amazing transformation at the Biggest Loser Ranch would earn me the reputation of being a master manipulator who would do anything to help my son win.

"Ron is one of the most competitive, cutthroat, manipulative players in this game," twenty-eight-year-old Kristin of the mother-and-daughter Purple Team would later say about me, during an episode in which the theme song from the movie *The Godfather* was played.

"I would be afraid for Filipe and Sione. They might find a horse head in their bed," said Tara, a twenty-three-year-old former model and Green Team member, referencing a scene from *The Godfather*.

"Keep your friends close, your enemies closer," I told Michael in our room as the drama intensified.

Michael later said, "My dad has played this game masterfully. He's playing chess. Everyone else is playing checkers."

From the start, I made no secret that I was controlling relationships in that house to position Michael to stay to the end. My secondary motive was to keep both of us there as long as possible, to lose weight and learn how to exercise and eat right.

However, the "game play" required to become the Biggest Loser had not crossed my mind in September 2008 when we'd first stepped onto the bus that took us to the Biggest Loser Ranch. Instead Michael and I were just awed that we had made our mark on the show's five-year history.

Michael was the youngest contestant ever. I was the sickest contestant ever. And we were part of the largest cast, with the heaviest contestants ever.

But would we be like contestants on prior episodes who worked out so diligently with the trainers? How sore and worn out would we feel, going from couch potatoes to fitness enthusiasts overnight? Would we be hungry?

As the bus barreled down the mountainous highway, we sat in the back row in our Brown Team T-shirts. The other twenty contestants were paired in matching-color T-shirts, and a camera crew was interviewing each team.

This was the first time we heard the other contestants' stories that would air on episode one. Even though we'd all been in the hotel for two weeks, we had never interacted with each other, except for brief introductions after learning we'd be coming to the ranch.

We had no idea if the ranch was a five-minute drive or a five-hour drive, so every freeway exit made us feel like excited kids asking, "Are we there yet?"

All we could think about was losing weight and staying at the ranch as long as possible. As fans of the show, we knew that every week at least one person was sent home.

If you've ever seen *The Biggest Loser: Couples*, you know that the goal is for each team to score the highest percentage of weight loss, not the total number of pounds lost.

The drama peaks at weekly weigh-ins, as a giant scoreboard lists the teams, the number of pounds lost, and the percentage of weight lost. At each weigh-in, at least two players fall below the yellow line on the scoreboard by having the lowest percentages of weight lost.

Those in jeopardy make the case for why they should stay, and the other contestants vote on who leaves. In the end, four finalists remain. The person with the largest percentage of weight loss is the Biggest Loser and wins $250,000.

As we sized up our competition on the bus, I prayed that that person would be Michael. The other teams were:

- **The Green Team:**   former models Tara from New York and Laura from Florida
- **The White Team:**   grandparents Jerry and Estella from Illinois
- **The Yellow Team:**   sisters Mandi and Aubrey from Idaho
- **The Blue Team:**   cousins Filipe and Sione from Arizona
- **The Orange Team:**   best friends Daniel and Dave from North Carolina
- **The Purple Team:**   daughter and mother Kristin and Cathy from Wisconsin
- **The Red Team:**   engaged couple Nicole and Damien from New York
- **The Black Team:**   brothers-in-law Blaine and Dane from Arizona

- **The Silver Team:**   best friends Joelle and Carla
                          from Michigan
- **The Pink Team:**   mother and daughter Helen
                          and Shannon from Michigan

The bottom line was that we were a busload of obese people with the same dream: to get thin and healthy thanks to this amazing opportunity of a lifetime.

I got worried at one point, when I realized that fifteen of the twenty-two people on the bus were under thirty years old. I was fifty-four. But Helen and Cathy were moms with grown kids, and Jerry and Estella were grandparents in their sixties. Did I have a fighting chance?

Finally, the bus drove through the regal-looking black and gold gates of the Biggest Loser Ranch.

"Oh my God!" people shrieked as we approached the Spanish-style building, with its terra-cotta roof and pale yellow stucco exterior. We all oohed and aahed, and stepped off that bus like we were in weight-loss nirvana. We thought we'd get to go to our rooms and get settled, but they took us straight to the 24 Hour Fitness gym!

We were so excited that we would work out with world-famous trainers Bob Harper and Jillian Michaels in that state-of-the-art facility.

"Oh my God, Michael," I said as we trudged up the trail to the gym. My knee was hurting like hell, but as we walked inside I was determined to push through the pain. "Can you believe it? It's the start of all of our new lives!"

"We can't get started fast enough," Michael said.

"This is it, home sweet home," said show host Alison Sweeney, greeting us as we looked around in awe at all the cardio machines, weights, and exercise contraptions.

"I want to win, Dad," Michael said, with more fire in his eyes than I'd ever seen. "I want to do everything I can to become the Biggest Loser."

I hugged him. "I'll do everything I can to help you do that."

"It is time for you to get your very first workout," Alison said, "and there's no better way to test what you're really made of than to ask you to do it alone. Because this first workout is without your trainers."

We looked at each other as if exclaiming, "What?" It was a hilarious scene as we fumbled around with the equipment.

"What do you do with these rubber-band straps?" I asked Michael.

Unbeknownst to us, Bob and Jillian were upstairs, watching us on a monitor. We were relieved and thrilled when they finally walked in.

But here was our first of many bittersweet moments on the ranch when disappointment obliterated euphoria. It happened as the contestants picked teams to work with each trainer.

Michael and I were chosen second to last. Standing there, feeling unwanted, I flashed back nearly fifty years to the pain and rejection of being the fat kid in gym class. Nobody wanted me on their team unless we were playing tug-of-war. I hated that Michael was feeling the same pain now—with cameras rolling.

It didn't help that the nine teams already picked were cheering and hugging, while we just stood there, trying to mask our dejected feelings. This was worse than gym class because even the other fat people didn't want us.

Finally, the mother-daughter Pink Team from Michigan picked us to join Bob's team.

As a viewer, I'd always loved Bob's "tough love" training style, so it was a thrill to meet him and know that he would transform me and my son into the men we were supposed to be.

The very first thing Bob said to me was, "Are you limpin'? Oh my God, I got a damaged guy already!"

We laughed, but the truth was that my knee *was* killing me. And looking around that gym, I was scared. How would I endure eight hours of daily exercise when I could barely walk? Geez, I had a permanent handicap sticker on my SUV back home, and someday soon I would need knee-replacement surgery.

Michael looked so eager; my stomach cramped with worry.

"Please, God, don't let me ruin this for him."

After that we had a vigorous workout with Bob and Jillian for a few hours. We couldn't wait to get to our rooms and collapse on our beds.

Michael and I lucked out with the spacious Brown Room. It was at the end of the hall, with windows on two sides and lots of sun, and it had really cold air-conditioning. For a heavy guy who sweats easily, that was great news in sunny California.

In our room, we'd soon learn to appreciate every precious minute of sleep. The first morning we awoke there, we were nearly paralyzed with pain. Every muscle in our bodies was sore. I thought, "Okay, I have to go to the bathroom, but I don't know if I'm gonna be able to stand up."

"I hurt from head to toe," Michael said from his twin bed.

"We have to push through the pain and hope our muscles get used to it," I said, trying to convince both of us.

Later that week what I saw at the Cedars-Sinai Medical Center would make me want to leap out of bed every day to stay as healthy as possible.

For a fat guy, it's bad enough to look in the mirror and see the evidence of your foodaholic lifetime. But thanks to the show, I had the rare opportunity to see the fat that was smothering my organs and engulfing my heart.

The show's physician, Dr. Rob Huizenga, an associate professor of clinical medicine at the University of California, Los Angeles, gave each contestant an extensive medical evaluation. The goal was to determine how obesity had ravaged our bodies.

After being stuffed into an MRI machine like a sausage, I was stunned by huge white patches of pure fat that showed up on the 3-D images of my abdomen. It was like someone had shoved giant scoops of lard inside my gut.

"It's just a huge, huge amount of fat," Dr. Huizenga said. "Your skin can't even take any more in, so it's depositing it around your liver and inside your abdomen and around your heart. And that's when some of the really dangerous things can start occurring."

That scared me to tears. All I could think about was that my sons would soon be facing the same death sentence.

I told myself, "We have to stay here and undo this damage. For me. For Michael. For Max at home."

I didn't know what it would take to make that happen. And I didn't care. Even if they called me the Godfather and the Hatchet Man.

Mike
Our Lives Depended on Staying on the Show

"You could die within five years."

That's what Dr. H told me after my first medical evaluation. Basically, if I kept gorging on fast food, eating 7,000 calories a day, never exercising, and gaining seventy-five pounds a year, I would keel over before finishing medical school. How ironic would that be?

Those six words from Dr. H were the biggest wake-up call I'd ever had. It made me believe that my food addiction was more lethal than smoking or drinking alcohol or doing drugs. Those habits took many years to kill; mine needed only five years.

My second reality check was stepping onto the giant scale for the first time on the show. This was not the first competitive weigh-in that would determine our status on the show; instead each contestant and team was being weighed to determine our starting weights prior to hitting the gym and learning how to eat low-calorie meals.

Wearing only shorts, I was so disgusted with exposing my sixty-five-inch belly on television. Twelve million Americans would be watching, along with people in ninety countries around the world. I was showing them the result of my secret binges, alone in my car, when I'd drive from one fast-food place to the next, stuffing down thousands of calories in a matter of minutes. I was a closet eater suddenly outed by choice as my feet hit that silver square and my weight flashed on the giant number display behind me: 388 pounds.

My five-foot-eleven frame was holding the weight of two large men combined. I was furious at myself for getting this way, so I channeled that rage into more intense workouts than I ever thought possible.

"One more!" Bob shouted as I pressed the barbell over my head, grimacing and dripping sweat. "There you go, Mikey! It's you and me!"

My first workout with Bob was the hardest thing I'd ever done. But I told myself, "I'm gonna win. I'm gonna be the Biggest Loser. I'm young. I'm strong. No one else can do what I can do."

That was my mentality from the moment I stepped onto the bus. Losing weight is all about what's going on in your mind. And I decided, "If I've been lucky enough to get this opportunity, then I have to take it all the way. And win."

I had psyched myself up to such a pitch that I wanted to

fast-forward to the finale and stand on the scale as the winner. I envisioned myself as a winner who had not only triumphed in the gym under Bob's training but had also learned how to eat in a healthy way to lose weight and maintain a thin body. I decided to keep that thought in my mind until I became the winner. Maybe it helped that I was eighteen, and I knew that under all these layers of fat a strong young man was just screaming to escape and make a positive impact on the world.

But despite all that confidence, walking into the weigh-in for the first episode was scary and intimidating. I thought, "This could be the moment when it's all over and we have to go home, still fat."

Like most things on the show, the first competitive weigh-in had a surprise twist: every team would send one member home; if the person who remained at the ranch did well, his or her teammate would be allowed to return. During this first weigh-in, that frightening prospect applied to everyone except the pair that won the weigh-in by losing the highest percentage of weight and the team that had won immunity at the challenge (Dane and Blaine).

That challenge involved all of us standing on a huge bridge at night in Los Angeles. At the center was an enormous mound of sand: 250,000 pounds. They said it symbolized the fact that we were standing between two lives—the unhealthy ones we were leaving behind, and the healthier ones in our future. The goal? To run up and over this mini-mountain of dirt as fast as we could.

I ran up and over it.

"C'mon, Dad!" I shouted as Dad struggled to walk and climb up the dirt.

Needless to say, we didn't win that challenge. But that didn't stop us from working superhard in the gym afterward. The first episode showed workouts and video clips of each team back at home. A camera crew had come to our house, prior to our trip to Los Angeles, to show us serving up spaghetti and meatballs in our kitchen; Dad and I shared our challenges and goals as part of the introductory video report. A similar video report profiled the other teams back in their hometowns, outlining their challenges and their goals.

The climax of episode one, of course, was the first weigh-in. I thought about it constantly; I was nervous beyond words. All I wanted was for me and Dad to lose enough weight to stay another week, and then all the way to the finale.

I knew from day one that if my dad ever got sent home, and I was there alone, I would snap. If he went home, I feared that he would never lose weight. I felt the same way about myself, but for Dad it was a more immediate issue of life or death. Even thinking about that for a split second made me believe that, alone at the ranch without him, I would become a maniac in the gym and a ruthless game player. I would be on a mission to win so that I could make my dad proud and miraculously inspire him to lose weight too. I needed him there to lose weight and get healthy, so he'd be around for years to come. This show had to be his saving grace. I saw our time on the ranch as the key to saving our lives.

For the first episode, we had been weighed to kick off the show and reveal just how high the numbers registered on the scale for our starting weights.

In total, the eleven couples weighed 3.5 tons!

Daniel, at age nineteen, was the heaviest contestant ever, at 454 pounds, with a prognosis that he might die before age thirty.

Carla, at thirty-nine, was the biggest woman ever on the show, weighing 379 pounds.

Jerry, at sixty-three, was the oldest contestant ever.

Tipping the scales at 388, I was the youngest contestant.

And Dad, starting at 430 pounds, was the show's sickest contestant ever.

After exercising with our trainers and learning how to cook and eat healthier in the kitchen, it was time for another weigh-in—the first official competitive weigh-in of the season, and the one that could get us sent home.

My whole body was shaking with nervousness as all the teams were weighed before me and Dad. When it was our turn, Alison said, "Gentlemen, in order to win this weigh-in, get above the yellow line, beat the Green Team, and stay on campus, you need to have lost more than forty-eight pounds."

I exhaled really hard because the pressure inside my body felt like I would explode. Behind me, the display showed 388, my starting weight.

Alison said, "Your current weight is . . ."

366!

I felt so happy—and shocked. I had lost twenty-two pounds in my first week! Here was my first taste of the bittersweet reality of being there. It felt amazing to lose way more weight than I'd ever been able to lose at home. But if Dad and I didn't lose enough weight in total, that's exactly where we'd be going. With that in mind, I couldn't fully celebrate my thrilling loss because I didn't know if Dad had lost the whopping twenty-six pounds necessary for us to win this weigh-in and keep both of us here.

"We have to stay," I repeated to myself. "We have to win. We have to become the Biggest Losers."

Dad's starting weight of 430 showed on the display behind him.

Alison said, "Your current weight is . . ."

The number 398 popped onto the screen, along with the pounds lost: 32.

"Oh my God! Amazing!"

We won! We won the very first weigh-in on the show by losing fifty-four pounds between us! That was the highest percentage of weight lost among the contestants.

I grinned. Standing between the scales, Dad and I shared a huge hug.

Our names rose to first place on the scoreboard—to the only spot above the yellow line—with a 6.6 percent weight loss.

And Dad set a record for the most weight anyone had ever lost in a single week. We didn't step down from the scales that night. We floated.

As a result of our weigh-in, we, along with the Black Team, which had won the immunity challenge, were the only teams that wouldn't get split up.

In the ominously red Elimination Room, we all sat at a long black table facing Alison. Behind us were eleven tall, lighted displays of the type that restaurants use to showcase cakes and pies. One case for each team, with the members' names glowing on top, over shelves of fake fattening foods like hunks of cheese or giant slices of cake. When a team was eliminated, its light would go dark.

"The Ron and Mike light will stay on until the finale," I decided. "We're going to shine."

But it was rough watching Shannon, of the Pink Team, decide that it was best for her mother, Helen, to stay. It was just as hard to see Cathy, the mom from another mother-and-daughter team, go home. I hoped that Kristin would do well enough for Cathy to return to the ranch in the near future.

Meanwhile, my heart was breaking for them, because they were like us: an obese parent and an obese kid, both fighting for a second chance at a normal life.

During the following week in the gym, I channeled all that sadness and fear into the weight machines and exercises. "I am the Biggest Loser," I repeated to myself when it hurt or I was tired. "Dad and I are staying until the finale. I am the Biggest Loser."

BECKY
We Had a Viewing Party Every Week

One day I was sitting in our dining room, which I use as a home office, when I happened to glance out the window. A light caught my eye: it was the big-screen TV inside our next-door neighbor's house.

And Michael appeared on the screen!

It was the most surreal moment of the whole season. I couldn't talk with them on the phone, e-mail, text, or write letters. Nothing.

But there was my son on TV, during a commercial promoting the show.

Every week eight or ten friends came over to watch the show with me and Max in the family room. I served healthy snacks like veggies and low-fat dip.

"There they are!" everybody cheered when Michael and Ron appeared. "Look! Look!"

It was so exciting to see our family on television. When they won the first weigh-in, we all went wild, cheering and jumping around. Here we were, in the room where we'd done so much eating while watching television, and now Michael and Ron were on the screen, shrinking before our very eyes.

I was so proud of Michael for losing weight. I would often think back to that moment in the kitchen when we first talked about him and Ron auditioning for the show. It had seemed like such a faraway dream. But now they were there, and it was changing their bodies and their lives.

When they first left, it felt like my husband and son had vanished into the Twilight Zone. Ron had called on Saturday, September 20, 2008, to say they were going to the ranch. After that we had no contact for three months. I couldn't watch them on TV because the show wouldn't air until January.

And we had to keep it all a secret! Even when Ron disappeared from the South Lyon City Council, and residents wanted to boot him off for good. We weren't allowed to tell anybody until December 12, when the commercial for season seven would air during the finale of season six.

All the while, I was a bundle of nerves, thinking about Ron's health and afraid that Michael might come home still heavy and no longer enrolled in college.

The unpredictability of the situation made it impossible to make plans. I wanted to visit my parents, especially because my dad's health was failing, but I was afraid to leave home in case Ron and Michael suddenly showed up.

Meanwhile, Max was going to the gym more often but still working at McDonald's and not eating right. I hoped that by watching Michael and Ron succeed, he would be inspired to do the same.

RON
From Hiding, into the Spotlight

My experience at the ranch was the opposite of how I'd lived my entire life. As a heavy guy, I'd spent years trying *not* to get noticed. I hated when strangers stared at me with disgust or pity, so I'd always tried to blend in and be invisible.

Now cameras were watching my every move, so people around the entire world would see everything I did!

"What the hell did I just get myself into?" I sometimes wondered.

On top of that, I had to do the most humiliating thing of all—step on a scale—on global TV! And then there were the workouts. For an overweight guy, the most intimidating place is the gym. That's where buff guys strut their stuff and show off how much weight they can lift. For an obese guy with bad knees, even the treadmill looks like a torture device.

"Geez, I'm 'the sickest contestant' ever on the show. How am I gonna do this?" I wondered.

I had to tell myself, "Stop it, Ron."

For all these years, it had been all about me and my addiction. Now everything would be about Michael and Max. If I was afraid or self-conscious or worried, I'd just have to suck it up and think about saving my sons.

And no one was more surprised than me when I realized that what I'd heard from so many people was true: after a few days you get used to the cameras and don't really think about them. You just focus on the next arm curl in the gym or the next challenge or the next vote in the Elimination Room.

Even though I'd watched the show for five years, I'd never thought about the people behind the cameras. You spend so much time with them that they feel like part of your family. You get to know whose wife is pregnant, who likes to play video games, and that kind of stuff. Being on the show also gave me a better understanding of all the things you don't see or realize while sitting on your couch at home watching every week.

For example, I never knew big boom microphones were swooping down over the contestants so viewers could hear what they were saying.

For me, what mattered most was what I was silently saying in my mind while praying. Growing up as a devout Catholic and attending parochial school, I drew on my faith to fuel me through the toughest moments, especially the weigh-ins.

Since our shorts had no pockets, I always wore a black wristband. At home I had cut the stitching open and inserted four

religious medals with special meaning for me: one of Father Sola-
nus Casey, a Capuchin priest from Detroit who may become
the first American saint; plus Our Lady of Confidence; Good
Saint Anne, who was Mary's mom and Jesus's grandmother; and
St. Joseph, Jesus's father. I had carried these medals in my wallet
since 1985. On the show, I wore that wristband unless I was in the
pool or the shower. During weigh-ins, I'd put my hand over the top
of it and pray that those saints would get us all the way to the finale.

I knew they were listening on the night of the first weigh-
in when Michael and I won with the highest percentage of
weight loss.

Mike
Eating to Live

Taco salad, white fish seasoned and grilled to perfection, and
corn tortilla wraps with cheese.

These were just some of the delicious, low-calorie creations
that Dad and I made in the huge gourmet kitchen at the ranch.
We both love to cook, and preparing healthy foods together was a
really awesome experience. If I started to wonder why we couldn't
have done this at home, I immediately stopped. I realized that it
was pointless to try to analyze the past and wish anything were
different. Of course I wish I had never become morbidly obese. Of
course I wish I could have exercised and eaten healthily at home so
my weight would not have approached four hundred pounds. But
that wasn't my story.

I felt like there, at the ranch, I was getting a chance to create
a new lifestyle. When I left, it was like I was starting over, fresh
from a crash course on how I could live a better life for decades
to come. And it was amazing to do that right alongside my dad.

"It's perfect," Dad said, standing at the restaurant-grade gas stove amid the yellow cabinets and checkered brown-and-white tile backsplash. He opened the aluminum foil just enough to allow a spicy waft of steam to rise up from the tilapia he'd cooked on the griddle.

"Mmm," I said. My muscles were burning and my stomach was gurgling with hunger after a fat-blasting workout with Bob in the gym. As odd as it sounds, the sensation of hunger was a new experience for me. For most of my life, I had disrupted the normal cycles of hunger: eat a balanced meal, get hungry a few hours later, eat another balanced meal, etc. Prior to this, I had no eating cycle; I ate so much and so frequently, for most of my waking hours (especially during my teen years), that I rarely felt hunger pangs. Here, though, eating three healthy meals and two snacks every day, and working out six or eight hours, I was revving my metabolism like never before.

Now I viewed healthy food as high-quality fuel my body could use to burn off all those chicken nuggets, pizzas, and chocolate chip cookies that had enlarged my fat cells. At home I was living to eat. Here, I was learning how to eat to live.

"I seasoned it with Mrs. Dash," Dad said as he served us each a plate with eight ounces of the white fish. Then he divided up a bag of frozen mixed vegetables, which he had steamed. We carried our plates into the dining room and enjoyed the meal with water. We had made a radical shift, but we were excited about the results, so we kicked into autopilot pretty quickly. Dad and I wanted nothing more than to finally lose weight there at the ranch. And eating smaller portions and lighter fare was the way to do that.

As closet eaters, we were relieved that the world didn't get to watch us eat. The kitchen and dining room were two of the few places at the ranch where cameras did not capture our every move. Sneaking food and eating in private was not an option in a kitchen shared by twenty-two contestants or a house wired with cameras. Dad had told me how comfortable he'd been among the other overweight people at Structure House. We felt that comfort with the other contestants, but here at the ranch there was an edge, because we were all competing for the Biggest Loser title and $250,000 prize.

Dad and I also had committed so strongly to making a dramatic transformation that we wanted to follow the show's regimen down to every last calorie.

But that didn't make us feel automatically comfortable eating in front of others. Fortunately, Dad and I had each other. Coming on the show made my very private obsession with food become a very public subject. I was just glad that cameras weren't watching me take every bite in the dining room.

So when you watch the show, you only see us eating at special events, like when celebrity chef Rocco DiSpirito cooked for winners of a challenge, and when some of us had that crazy night at a luxury spa while Dad made filet mignon for several other contestants back at the ranch.

So how did we know what to eat on most days?

When we arrived in September, Dr. H told each of us how many calories we should eat each day. The kitchen was stocked with fresh fruits, vegetables, lean meats, healthy grains, and low-fat dairy products. But we had to plan our own menus. At first it seemed bizarre to set twenty-two obese people free in a kitchen and expect us to make low-calorie meals. I mean, our inability to eat healthy meals and small portions was the reason we were all obese. But I loved how we were forced to sink or swim. We very quickly figured out how to calculate what we could eat within our daily calorie allotments. Fortunately, Dad's experience at Structure House had taught him how to plan healthier meals, so he drew on that knowledge and taught me.

Why didn't we do this at home?

Dad wasn't ready. I wasn't ready. But now we were. Plus, we had no choice. We had our eyes on the prize, and in order to win we had to put vegetables, lean protein, and some healthy carbs into our bodies every day. That was part of the amazing learning process at the ranch.

The trainers gave each of us a book of calorie counts that listed every food you could imagine. The kitchen was also stocked with *Biggest Loser* cookbooks, and the trainers told us to weigh and measure everything so we could accurately count every calorie. Beyond that, we were pretty much on our own. No trainers or nutritionists stood in the kitchen and said, "You should eat this, not that." But Bob periodically showed up, offering guidance.

"Eat every four hours," Bob told us. "Eat a protein and a starch at every meal and snack. Make sure your calories are spread out through the day."

With this information, I gave myself a crash course on counting calories with the healthy food provided in the kitchen. Dr. H told me that I needed 1,800–2,000 calories every day to become the Biggest Loser. It was shocking to realize that I could actually eat a large volume of food and stay within my daily allowance of calories. It was also mind-blowing to discover that my typical lunch at McDonald's equaled my entire daily calorie count.

My biggest aha! moment was realizing that losing weight is really just a math game. The key is calories in, calories out, and how you process those calories. Just like Mom had been showing me every day for years.

Duh!

That's the clinical explanation. My relationship with food, however, was totally emotional. At the ranch, I replaced that horrible cycle of food-fat-food with new outlets for my emotions: pumping iron. Running five miles every morning on the beautiful

Presidential Mile, which wound through the rugged mountainous terrain. Boxing. And doing calisthenics.

I was shocked to discover how phenomenal I felt after exercising. My mind was clear and my body felt alive and energized. It was also incredible to eat a meal and not feel stuffed or nauseous. Dad's dieting experience and culinary skills helped us write our daily menus. If we needed something special, like shrimp, the show's grocery team would go shopping.

Our typical breakfast was three to four egg whites with turkey bacon and two corn tortillas wrapped around fat-free feta cheese with hot sauce.

For lunch we'd have a bunless six-ounce burger made from 97 percent fat-free beef, an apple, and vegetables. Green beans are my favorite. I only like cooked vegetables, and I refuse to eat Brussels sprouts. I've never eaten one; they just look weird.

I became very innovative when it came to packing flavor into low-fat foods. In fact, I became the yogurt king, using it to make ranch dressing and steak sauce.

"Hey Mike," another contestant would say, "I need some of your spicy sour cream."

It wasn't really sour cream. It was a creation that I made from nonfat yogurt and Mexican spices. We used it on our low-calorie taco salad: crushed, baked tortilla chips on lettuce with spicy, low-fat turkey or beef.

Sometimes we'd snack on an apple and some almonds, a Fiber One Bar, or a whey-protein shake.

Bob and Jillian described our eating as "clean." That meant nothing processed or fried and no refined sugars. Instead we ate wholesome foods like vegetables, lean meats, and fruits in their original state.

At the beginning, the contestants shared this great camaraderie about being there to lose weight. Sometimes one person would even volunteer to cook for a small group. Fortunately, we all ate at different times. It would have been impossible for twenty-two people to cook simultaneously.

But I wondered if the competitive aspect of "the game" would eventually play out among the eleven teams in the kitchen.

It wasn't like someone poured fattening butter on your fresh fruit when you weren't looking. But if you saw a competitor cooking with a lot of oil, you sure didn't say anything about it. That was their choice, and if they fell below the yellow line as a result, for us that would mean one less competitor.

More than anything, I was actually in competition with myself. My new consciousness about food and exercise made me furious about abusing my body for all those years. In middle school, and especially high school, I'd been old enough to know better. Mom and Weight Watchers had taught me how to eat low-calorie meals. But I hadn't used that information. Now I hated that I'd had the knowledge but not the willpower.

There at the ranch, with every painful push-up or heart-pumping sprint on the treadmill, I was undoing the damage. I told myself, "I can't change the past. I can only control the future. I will be the Biggest Loser."

RON
The Game Master Is Born Below the Yellow Line

If the first weigh-in was heaven, the fourth weigh-in was hell.

I lost seven pounds; Michael lost nine.

At home we would have thrown a party to celebrate such an incredible feat. On *The Biggest Loser*, our combined sixteen-pound weight loss threatened to send us home.

For the first time, our competitors would decide whether to send me and Michael back to Michigan for good or spare us and boot the Orange Team off the ranch.

"When I saw the sixteen pounds," Michael said during a nighttime interview outside the gym, "I felt like I failed my dad, I failed my team, I failed myself, and there was nothing else, just, I failed."

Michael was crying. My heart was pounding, and my mind was spinning a million miles a minute, wondering: "How can I work this game to keep us on top? How can I convince these people to vote for us no matter what? How can I make sure that this never happens again, and if it does, how can I develop an alliance to protect us?"

I had already befriended everyone. Given my age and disabilities, I knew I was viewed as a nonthreat by the younger, stronger contestants. Being unable to excel in the challenges helped cement this image.

I was a father figure at the ranch, and when I spoke people listened. So I decided that if we weren't kicked off that night, after the fourth weigh-in, I would cultivate that image; I would never do or say anything to make people feel threatened by me. I would make people feel that I had their back, that we were on their side, and that our loyalty would be their safety net if they ever fell below the yellow line.

There's power in numbers. The higher the number of alliances, the greater your chances for staying on the ranch.

While I was figuring all this out, my son was still standing there at the weigh-in, crying.

I realized that I'd failed him. I should have worked out harder or done something to secure our place. "If we get to stay," I promised myself, "I will. With gusto."

I only felt worse when Alison told the other teams, "This is a difficult decision. You'll be deciding between father and son and best friends. You have one hour to make your decision."

Michael and I both hugged Bob, wondering if this was a final good-bye. I had lost sixty pounds; Michael had lost forty-nine. If we went back home now, after one month at the ranch, we'd fall back into our bad habits. Michael was no longer enrolled in college. With no school and no job, he'd have nothing to do but eat. The disappointment of losing would drive us to binge exponentially; we'd both be bigger than ever in a matter of weeks.

"No. That cannot happen," I prayed. "Please, God, please."

I prayed hard as we joined the other contestants to walk through the crisp nighttime air back to the house. We all gathered in the dining room.

During prior eliminations, I'd always considered who needed to be at the ranch to lose weight. Who had the support at home to make it happen? Who didn't? But that didn't work this time. Because we were up against nineteen-year-old Daniel, the heaviest contestant in *Biggest Loser* history, and his best friend, nineteen-year-old Dave, who had started at 393 pounds.

Both Daniel and Michael needed to be there just as desperately. In order to stay, we had to plead our case as if our lives depended on it—because ultimately they did. I needed to tug the heartstrings of every person in that room so that they would never write "Ron" or "Mike" on those color-coded elimination cards.

"As a dad, I feel like I failed my son," I said sadly, my voice cracking. Most of the women, especially Mandi, were crying. "I should have done better. I mean, I want to be here. I need to be here. My son needs to be here. I don't want to go, but you guys vote with your heart. But I want to stay and my son needs to stay."

Helen and Tara were crying; Cathy—who had since returned

to the ranch because her teammate and daughter, Kristin, was doing well—buried her face in her hands. Filipe and Sione teared up. I prayed that their sympathy would result in enough votes to keep us.

Blaine and Dane, who were on Jillian's team with Dan and Dave, looked sympathetic, but I assumed their loyalty would lie with the Orange Team.

"It's my job to protect him," I said, "and I didn't do it very well this week, and I'm sorry."

Michael, who was standing against the wall and crying, said, "It's both our fault."

"All I can ask is that you don't vote my son off this place," I said, my voice quaking. "Keep him. Kick me to the curb, but keep him."

I was speaking from my heart, with 100 percent sincerity, and it sparked a crying fest in that dining room.

Next Daniel pled the Orange Team's case but didn't get the tearful reaction that I had received. Then Dave said his commitment was to the program but his heart wasn't in it, and that he felt "trapped" on the ranch. That rubbed everybody wrong.

And I knew we would stay.

But first we'd have to endure some terrifying moments in the Elimination Room. Three of Jillian's team members voted for us to leave. Three of Bob's team members voted for us to stay. The Blue Team—Sione and Filipe—held the power to keep us or cast us out.

After a tearful statement about missing his wife and kids, Filipe lifted the silver dome to reveal a card that said: "Dan and Dave."

That's when Alison said, "Dan, Dave, with four votes you have been eliminated." Then she spoke words that Michael and

I never wanted to hear: "I'm sorry to tell you, you are not the Biggest Loser. It's time for you to go."

Somber-looking Michael rubbed Dan's shoulder. We didn't show our excitement because it was a sad moment for Dan and Dave. But inside we were ecstatic. We would stay!

This had been a bit too close for comfort, though. From that night on, this sickest contestant was on a crash course to learn the best "game play" ever to occur on *The Biggest Loser*.

And so the Game Master was born.

CHAPTER 10

/ # MIKE AND RON

Fighting to the Final Four

Mike
Reality Strikes below the Yellow Line, Again

I was eating fewer calories than I could ever remember doing. I was busting my butt in the gym. My body was responding to the program, and I was shrinking. Fast.

But the reality was that my dad wasn't. He was fifty-four years old, with a slower metabolism and two bad knees.

And it showed on the scale.

At the weigh-in for episode five, we fell below the yellow line for a second week in a row. That forced us to endure the gut-wrenching ordeal of being up for elimination. Again.

Whoomp!

It was like the grim reality of our situation slammed me in the chest.

I lost nine pounds.

Dad lost four.

"I was hoping for a better number than that," Dad said on the scale, looking devastated.

Bob looked so disappointed. "It was like a punch in the stomach," he said during an interview outdoors. "Oh, man, as bad as I feel, he's definitely feeling worse."

As I stood on the scale, rage shot through me. It wasn't fair that I was working so hard, and that we both wanted to be here, yet it wasn't good enough.

A split second later, I realized that it wasn't my dad's fault. He was trying. He wanted to do the work to keep us at the ranch, but it was physically impossible.

So far in the challenges, he'd lagged far behind or sat out altogether. During the first week, he could barely climb the mountain of sand on the bridge in downtown Los Angeles. For the second week, he stayed on the boat while I came in fifth in the ocean-mountain race on kayaks and a foot trail. In the third week, Dad was almost immediately eliminated for stepping on the giant metal jump rope and breaking the Styrofoam, because he couldn't jump. I hung in there for that challenge, but it was rough. It was 95°F that day, and Tara won after two hours and nineteen minutes with 1,030 jumps. Dad could never do that. *I* couldn't even do that.

For the fourth week's challenge, which aired during Super Bowl week, NFL quarterback Kurt Warner joined us on a football field. We had to run back and forth to eliminate players by putting footballs in bins. Again Dad could barely walk, much less run. And the current week's challenge involved the difficult task of climbing over and under a pipe while unwrapping rope.

All of this flashed through my mind at the weigh-in as the other teams stepped on the scales. The anxiety of wondering whether they would score lower percentages of weight loss was maddening.

In my mind, everything was a giant question mark. I'd been

so confident after winning the first weigh-in. Going home after five weeks would kill me.

No! I decided.

I already felt that I had to carry our team as the younger, stronger member. But the pressure that night was almost unbearable. I was accomplishing things that five weeks ago I never thought possible—9 pounds in one week? Amazing. I'd already lost 58 pounds, weighing in that night at 330. But I couldn't feel happy because we could still lose out on the greatest opportunity of our lives.

It wasn't fair, but it was reality.

This was a competition. A team effort. And our thirteen pounds equaled a 1.83 percent weight loss, which pushed us below the yellow line. In contrast, the Green Team lost twenty-five pounds, for a weight loss of 4.84 percent.

The silver lining on this ominous cloud was that the Silver Team fell below the yellow line with us. Everyone loved Carla, who was just back on the ranch after her thirty days at home. After giving it 100 percent, she lost nine pounds that week and was ecstatic. But her friend Joelle lost zero. Zero pounds! Everyone, including Bob, believed she wasn't trying and didn't even care.

"I've never seen Bob this mad," Jillian said after he yelled at Joelle in the gym when she was giving up. We all had to do extra sprints on the treadmills because she was slacking. We were totally baffled how someone could blow the chance to work out with world-class trainers in a multimillion-dollar gym. Especially when Carla was depending on her to stay.

"Brown Team, Silver Team," Alison said at the end of the weigh-in, "this is not your first trip below the yellow line for either of you."

My stomach was in knots.

It seemed like an obvious choice between us and the Silver Team because Joelle had disappointed everybody. But at the ranch, you expect the unexpected. So Dad and I had to plead our case. Again.

We all went into the living room, where Dad and I sat on the couch. Ironically, the drama that exploded was all about teamwork.

"This is not about *you*!" Carla shouted at Joelle. "This is about *us*!"

Carla cried, and you could see the angst on the faces of the Pink Team, the Blue Team, the Yellow Team, the Purple Team, the Black Team, and the Green Team.

But for me, Carla's words echoed some of my thoughts. It was worse, though, because Dad was trying and cared with all his heart.

"I'm sorry," Carla told Joelle, crying. "I really want to be here. And this is the second time I put my fate in your hands, and twice you failed me, twice!"

My gut twisted as Carla's pain mirrored my own frustration.

"I'm trying to work out double and as hard for the both of us," Carla continued, "because I knew you wouldn't lose enough weight to keep us here."

I buried my head in my hands, fighting back tears.

"Because of my teammate," Carla said, "I have to suffer. And that's really messed up. It really is."

I could never say anything like that out loud, to the group or to Dad. We both knew that was our reality. The difference was that I couldn't stay mad because his mind and heart were totally committed. I prayed that this would inspire the other teams to vote for us.

When it was my turn, I said, "What I have to say is, words are cheap in this house and actions speak. You see us in the gym every single day as long as you are. We're in this 100 percent. I want to be here. I'm trying my best, and this week it wasn't good enough."

Then Dad's voice was soft with sadness and desperation, and his eyes were pleading with everyone.

"I asked you last week not to send my son home, and I'm going to ask you again. Please don't send us home. One hundred percent of this team wants to be here. One hundred percent. And I hope you guys vote that way."

In the elimination room, we all faced Alison at the long black table. One person from each team sat in front of the fate-defining silver plate with its domed cover hiding the vote written on a card. Dad sat; I stood.

"We've given you chances again and again," Tara said before casting the fourth vote that would send the Silver Team home. The Pink Team, the Yellow Team, and the Blue Team had already cast three votes against Joelle and Carla.

"It's time to just stop with the second chances," Tara said.

Relief overwhelmed me. But those words "second chances" hit me hard. This was a second chance for us. What if we needed a third chance, and the other teams got sick of taking pity on us?

I was scared as hell.

Especially when Bob told me to eat *more*.

"The Brown Team is not going to be below the yellow line," Bob said emphatically. "Two weeks in a row, you guys were below the yellow line. Enough!"

He added that if we bombed another weigh-in, he would have met the team he couldn't help. And that would drive him crazy.

But his solution made *me* feel crazy.

He said I had cut my calories so drastically that my body was holding on to weight. Apparently our bodies are programmed to slow their metabolism—and thus fat burning and weight loss—when we drastically cut back on food. It's like some instinctual mechanism from prehistoric times; our bodies think food is scarce, so they store fat so we don't starve to death. To combat this, Bob told me to consume more calories by eating bigger portions of the fish, poultry, yams, and other vegetables that I was already eating. He said eating more would stimulate my metabolism. But my instincts were telling me that eating more was the wrong approach. I was so desperate to keep losing weight fast that I believed the only way to succeed was to eat as few calories as possible.

But Bob was the expert trainer. I had to trust him.

Amazingly, eating more actually worked! I lost thirteen pounds at the next weigh-in. It seemed like every week I was learning something new about nutrition, fitness, and weight loss. Who knew that adding calories would help me lose weight? Shocking and thrilling all at once, this rejuvenated my hope that I could become the Biggest Loser.

BECKY
It Was Hard to Watch the Challenges

I cringed every time Michael and Ron struggled through a challenge. When they had to find the keys to the gym by running up and down a mountain trail during episode seven, I could hardly watch.

I could only imagine how much Ron's knees were hurting as he crept at a turtle's pace up that trail, under the blazing California sun. Even worse, he'd have to exercise outdoors all week if neither he nor Michael found the gym key from a board holding dozens of keys at the top of the hill. Michael ran back and forth, trying multiple keys in the padlocks that were chaining the gym doors shut.

It pained me that Michael was working doubly hard to make

up for Ron's handicap, and that Ron must have felt guilty for putting that burden on Michael.

Amazingly, Michael found the key!

"I gotta go get my dad!" he exclaimed, dashing up the hill to spare Ron from the painful hike. I loved that Michael was always thinking about how he could help his dad.

Likewise, it was comforting that Ron was at the ranch to run interference for Michael when they were below the yellow line. Even though I hated the Game Master persona, I understood why Ron was doing it, and I was thrilled that, so far, it was working to keep them there.

Mike
I Was in the Hot Seat Again

During the eighth week, Dad and I were separated onto different teams. The original teammates were split up and divided between Jillian's Black Team and Bob's Blue Team. I was on the Black Team while Dad was on the Blue Team over the course of several episodes. Even worse, we faced an insane challenge: ride stationary bicycles for twenty-four hours straight!

The team that rode the most miles would win a three-pound advantage at the next weigh-in and custom Trek bikes for each member.

My team, the Black Team, won by riding 301.9 miles. That set a precedent for victory against the Blue Team, which was Dad, Cathy, Kristin, Aubrey, Mandi, and Dane.

My teammates were Tara, Laura, Filipe and Sione, and Helen. I went with the flow as far as this Black Team versus Blue Team stuff was concerned. But during the weigh-in for the ninth week, the surprise twist put outrageous pressure on me.

"Tonight's weigh-in is unlike anything we've ever done on *The Biggest Loser*," Alison said when we arrived in blue and black T-shirts for the weigh-in.

"You will not be weighing in against each other," she said. "You will be weighing in with each other."

We all looked at each other like, "What?"

"You all are about to have the chance to win immunity for everyone," Alison said. "If you lost a pound a day for the last week, all of you are guaranteed one more week on campus. You have to lose a combined total of seventy-seven pounds."

My heart was pounding in my chest. I was the last person to step on the scale.

"We have one person left to weigh," Alison said. "Mike, it all comes down to you."

I stepped up to the scale, trembling with terror.

"In order for everyone to have immunity, for one more week on campus," Alison said, "you need to have lost more than nine pounds."

I'd never felt so stressed. I'd had three weeks of double-digit weight loss in a row. This stressed me out because I was afraid I couldn't continue to lose at such a fast rate. I worried that my weight loss would plateau, that it would hover at a certain weight. I had heard from trainers and other contestants that plateaus were a normal and expected part of weight loss. And that scared me.

"I don't feel that I've lost weight this week," I said, my face tense. The week before, I'd weighed in at 297. That meant the scale now had to show 287 maximum.

"If I don't lose ten pounds," I said, "I'm killing two people's dreams. That feeling is horrible. That's way too much pressure for me."

Alison asked how I was doing.

"Not good," I answered, adding that I was "a neurotic mess" and that the pressure wasn't helping.

Alison said, "Your weight is . . ."

"To Be Continued" flashed across the TV screen when this episode aired. I had no idea that viewers would have to wait to see if I'd lost enough to save two people from going home. Fortunately, I didn't have to wait.

The display flashed minus eleven.

Yes!

My weight loss kept everybody at the ranch for another week.

And I passed the 100-pound mark! In three months, I had lost 102 pounds.

"I am the Biggest Loser . . ."

Max
I Was Still Eating Badly

The holidays were coming, and I hadn't seen my brother or dad in months. Mom had decorated the house for Christmas, and she always did a pretty job. But I didn't feel like celebrating. The house was so quiet without Dad and Michael. I was happy for them because they were still losing weight in California. I couldn't imagine how they'd look; I'd only known them as obese.

It felt like they were far away, on an adventure into a new life, while I was still at home, stuck in my old, bad habits. I was still scarfing down thousands of calories every day, thanks to my job at McDonald's and frequent trips through other fast-food drive-throughs. Having the car all to myself made it even easier to eat whenever I wanted.

Unfortunately, I didn't make as many trips to the gym as I'd hoped. It was so easy to blow off my workouts by doing home-work, hanging out with friends, working, or playing video games. Sometimes I did go to the gym—definitely more than before Dad and Michael left—but since I was still eating so badly, I was still huge.

Without Michael—my eating buddy and video game partner—I had too much time to think. I hated imagining that he and Dad would come home skinny, and since I had failed to slim down while they were gone, I would be the only fat one in the fam-ily. That thought would make me eat to forget about all the bad feelings: missing them, wishing I were thin, and hating that I still weighed nearly four hundred pounds as a high school junior.

While thinking about my life, I've never been one to get deep and analytical about things. For me, it's pretty simple. I feel a certain way, I do certain things, and that becomes my life. I don't like to sit around trying to figure out the psychological motiva-tions for stuff. I had no desire to look back on my childhood and play a blame game about why I was fat. That wouldn't change anything.

All I could do was look forward and wish for the motivation to finally take over so I could stick to a diet and exercise plan.

Even though Mom was the queen of low-calorie eating, I just couldn't get myself to start or stick to a plan. If Dad and Michael had been at home and in the kitchen every day making salads and grilled chicken like Mom, then it would have been easy for me to join their plan.

Of course Mom was trying to help. But after that first healthy shopping trip, I went back to fast food, chips, and huge portions. In fact, I weighed more than Michael when he was fifteen. He and Dad were living a dream in California; I was still stuck in my nightmare where I couldn't stop eating and gaining weight. And soon TV cameras would be at our house to expose my depressing situation to the whole world.

BECKY
The Happiest Moment of My Life

I hadn't spoken to Michael for more than three months. It was December 20, 2008, and Ron and Michael were coming home for Christmas. We had to take down all the holiday decorations because camera crews for *The Biggest Loser* would be filming the father-and-son team's homecoming, and the segment would air months after the holiday season.

I had no idea what they would look like, because the seventh season wouldn't air until the following month, January. I was amazed and grateful that they'd lasted this long.

It was exciting but stressful as we got everything ready. Excitement buzzed in the house. Forty or fifty friends and family members gathered to await Ron and Mike's grand arrival home. The producers had them all sign releases saying they agreed to appear on the show. My mind was spinning. How would Ron look? How would Michael look? I couldn't even imagine. But I was thrilled that they'd made it this far.

Max was in good spirits, joking with his grandfather about who'd be the first to cry when Ron and Michael came through the door. Michael's high school girlfriend stood near the front door with me and Max.

With the cameras rolling, Ron walked in—ninety-five pounds slimmer!

The house exploded with cheers. His hair was long and he had shrunken to the size he was when we left Structure House.

"If you think I look great," Ron said, "you should see your son!"

The producers had hidden Michael in the laundry room. He opened the door and popped his face and his hands out, as if to say, "Here I am!" He wore a brown shirt with a trendy logo, jeans, and white loafers. His hair was spiky, and I'd never seen such a huge, bright smile on his face.

The sight of him was so shocking that everyone was stunned silent. My heartbeat pounded in my ears.

"Oh my God!" I shrieked, bursting into tears as everyone went wild with cheers for Michael.

All I could do was stare at my son, who looked so stunningly different. I'd seen Ron lose weight before. But never Michael. His double chin and chubby cheeks were gone. His belly had deflated. And excitement twinkled in his eyes like I'd never seen.

He was 110 pounds slimmer in just three months.

I ran up and grabbed him. "Michael, you look amazing!"

That was the happiest moment of my life. Everyone in the house cheered as the cameras captured it all.

But in an instant, it became one of the worst moments of my life.

Max sobbed.

The producers thought he was crying tears of joy.

The house was silent again, except for Max's uncontrolled crying.

It was horrible.

"Poor child," a friend whispered.

Grandmas sobbed. Friends choked back tears. Sadness swept through the crowd as everyone's heart just broke for him. Michael's amazing moment had turned somber as he tried to comfort his brother. My overwhelming joy for Michael became inexpressible sadness for Max.

Max
The Worst Time of My Life

I stood in the kitchen, crying out of control. It was like pure misery shooting out of my mouth, and it sounded like a howl. I had never felt worse. My whole body was shaking as Dad and Michael tried to comfort me.

"It's okay, Max," Dad said, "this will happen for you too."

But nothing they said could fix the fact that they were shrinking and I was still nearly four hundred pounds. Seeing Michael, especially, made me feel like a failure. He was doing what we both wanted to do. But I was still home, going to school, working at McDonald's, stuck in our old habits.

I had thought I could lose weight while they were gone, but I couldn't. I'd gone to the gym more, but I was still eating thousands of extra calories every day. I didn't know how to be any different. Of course as I stood there crying like a baby in the kitchen I told myself that, from now on, I would change. But I knew that wouldn't happen. It never did. I just couldn't do it by myself.

I hated that the cameras were on me as I cried my heart out. I hated that everyone in the whole house was pitying me. And all the people who were going to watch this episode would also be sobbing over poor Max.

Every time I looked at Michael, I was happy for him, but I almost felt betrayed. He was my best friend. And he had been just as big as me. Now that guy was gone. I felt alone. Looking at Dad made it worse. All my life I'd wanted to be just like him. I was now, but he was changing too.

"I have to change. Now. But I don't think I can."

That thought only made me sob harder.

Mike
I Paid Max to Quit McDonald's

After the cameras were gone, and Dad and I had adjusted to being home, I had a talk with Max in the family room.

"If you quit McDonald's, I'll pay you the same amount of money you would be making," I promised. *The Biggest Loser* was paying me and my dad a hundred dollars a day, each, for the whole time we were on the show. For an eighteen-year-old kid, seven hundred dollars a week was a lot of cash, and I couldn't think of a better way to invest it than in my little brother's success.

Working around fries and burgers would make it impossible for Max to lose weight by himself.

"You can use the time that you'd be working to go to the gym," I encouraged.

Max nodded through tears. "Thanks, Michael. That'll work. I can do that. I want to be just like you."

That day, I went to McDonald's with Max, and he quit his job there.

I hoped this would help Max for now, and that someday he'd also get the chance of a lifetime that Dad and I had right now. Perhaps he could someday be on *The Biggest Loser*. Seeing him, and coming home to the "scene of the crime" where I had developed such horrible eating habits, made me realize how dramatically I had changed. I felt like a new person, one whose brain was being reprogrammed to think about food in a whole new way.

But joining my family and our friends at our favorite restaurant, the South Lyon Hotel, was still tough. *Biggest Loser* cameras captured the temptation as I ate a salad while sitting between two pizzas. They smelled so good, and I knew I could eat an entire one by myself, because I'd done it so many times before.

"I am the Biggest Loser," I told myself. "I will never be that obese guy who would eat four plates of fried fish and fries in this very restaurant."

So instead of reaching for a slice, I dipped my fork onto my vinaigrette salad dressing and speared another mouthful of salad.

"I never thought I'd see my son dip his fork in salad dressing!" Mom exclaimed. She was ecstatic because that was a trick that I'd seen her do a million times.

Still, it was terrifying. With one split-second decision, I could do major damage to that pizza in front of me. The ranch is a very controlled environment. You can't just leave and get a pizza, and you have to follow the schedule of workouts, challenges, and weigh-ins.

At home food was everywhere. I was tempted, but all I could think about was stepping back on that scale when I'd be back at the ranch after just one week at home. I still had a lot of weight to lose, but I was realizing that this would never be easy. "Even if I become the Biggest Loser, I'll have to work like crazy the rest of my life to keep the weight off."

That was my reality. Period. It made me mad, because I wanted to think that something in my brain would just click and I would robotically want to eat right and exercise every day. Wrong!

At the same time, seeing Max as big as I was when I left for the show reinforced my determination to keep losing weight, keep it off, and help him. As I considered all this, my thoughts were abruptly interrupted when Dad and I learned—via Alison on a DVD delivered to our door—that we'd have to run a half marathon while we were home.

I was thrilled that the training and the actual event would burn tons of calories. But running 13.1 miles scared the hell out of me. Could I run for that long? And how would Dad get through it?

Fortunately, our training was a good way to get Max out to walk with us. Dad and I walked as much as possible, and I ran. Most people spend months training for a marathon; we didn't have that luxury. I hoped that the exercise we'd been doing at the ranch would help us power through what sounded like a grueling ordeal. If I was dreading it for myself, then it must have sounded like a nightmare for Dad.

Since it was December in Michigan, we did the half marathon at an indoor track. Dad walked four miles in about two hours, but he was in so much pain that he couldn't finish. I finished and felt great about it. Just a few months before, running around the block would have been practically impossible at my size. So the fact that I did it was a huge confidence booster. My time didn't matter; I woke up the next morning thinking, "I did it!"

All that running paid off back at the ranch. The weigh-in revealed that I lost eight pounds at home; Dad lost ten and won immunity. He also passed the hundred-pound mark.

This was a huge jolt of confidence. We'd returned to the scene of the crime—home—and actually lost weight.

RON
The Sickest Contestant Goes to the ER

It was episode twelve, and we were on a NASCAR racetrack after pulling cars attached to harnesses on our bodies. I actually pulled the car despite the pain in my knees. Michael was in the lead, pulling his car around the track faster than the other contestants.

But when it was over, I knew something was wrong. I just didn't feel right. Then I went blind.

"Michael, I can't see," I said. "You gotta hold me up."

I was sure I would keel over on the racetrack. It was blazing hot as the California sun soaked into the black asphalt and radiated back up on us.

I was terrified, not just of passing out, but of doing so on camera. Would I get sick and have to leave the show? What would happen to Michael? My thoughts raced a mile a minute as I held on to Michael's arm.

The irony was that I loved NASCAR. I loved cars and watching races. For my fortieth birthday, I had received an autographed size 10X jacket autographed by Mario Andretti. So Michael and I had hauled ass in the challenge to win a trip to watch a real NASCAR race, and it was a thrill to meet NASCAR champion Clint Bowyer.

But now, suddenly, my health took a turn. I had never felt worse.

Cameras were still filming because Tara—who had pulled ahead of Michael to win the challenge—got to take a ride in a sleek yellow racecar with Clint. The last thing I wanted was to collapse on camera, like "oldest contestant" Jerry during the first hour at the ranch.

We had just had a weigh-in, and I'd lost ten pounds and won immunity, so Michael and I were both happy. But he looked terrified as he held me up. I prayed that I could stay conscious until this thing was over. Fortunately, I started feeling better.

But a day or two later, I was walking the Presidential Mile when suddenly it felt like someone was standing on my chest. I was dizzy and having heart palpitations. I couldn't catch my breath.

"God, please don't let me drop dead out here alone."

That was not how I wanted to leave the ranch.

I feared that after all those years of abusing my body, a combination of the stress of exercise and worry about being able to stay at the ranch were giving me a heart attack. Poor Michael was worried enough about me already.

I made it to Sandy, the medic, and told him my symptoms. My chest was hurting where I'd worn the harness to pull the car on the racetrack, so I hoped that was the culprit. But I also told him that I'd been passing black stool, which usually signaled internal bleeding.

He called am ambulance, which rushed me to the hospital before I could tell Michael what was going on.

Dr. Huizenga called a specialist at Cedars-Sinai Hospital. Cedars-Sinai is one of the three hospitals in America with a high-tech scope that descends through the throat to search for intestinal distress. They had a 10 percent chance of finding the culprit. But voilà! They found two ulcers in the part of my stomach that was blocked off by my gastric bypass surgery.

On a monitor, they showed me ulcer number one: a red circle with a dark indention at the center. Ulcer number two was a white circle. It was healing after bursting open and bleeding. I'd had scopes done before, but doctors could never find the problem.

Dr. H said I was one lucky guy. This ruled out a heart attack; blood loss had caused the dizziness. That was the good news. The bad news? They pumped me with thirteen pounds of blood and fluid over three days in the hospital.

No surprise, I fell below the yellow line at the next weigh-in. Meanwhile, Michael lost eleven pounds, becoming the Biggest Loser for the week.

Here's where the Game Master ruled.

All along I'd been building alliances and strategizing about how these relationships could work to keep me and Michael on the ranch. Early on, Cathy and I had made a pact to put our children first and sacrifice ourselves if necessary. Michael and I adored Cathy's daughter, Kristin, who began the show at 360 pounds.

We had also allied with the Blue Team, cousins Sione and Filipe, who, like Cathy and Kristin, were original members of Bob's team with us. We decided that the old Bob's team would stick together and eliminate the old Jillian's team. It worked; we eliminated everybody but Tara.

As the teams whittled down by episodes thirteen and fourteen, an "every man for himself" mentality set in. Only one person would become the Biggest Loser and win that $250,000 prize.

During eliminations, the question was, "Who's the biggest threat?" rather than "Who really needs to be here to lose weight?"

For me, anybody who was a threat to Michael needed to leave. That's why, the week before, when Filipe fell below the yellow line, I didn't vote for him. But he felt betrayed.

This week, before the elimination, he told me I'd be "fine." But Filipe voted against me, as did Sione and Helen. Fortunately, Tara, Laura, Kristin, and Mike voted against Nicole, who went home.

I stayed.

"I'm like the contestant that won't leave," I told Bob, who was amazed that I'd made it through yet another elimination.

But the tension was as thick as molasses. When I walked back into the house after Filipe and Sione failed to eliminate me, the look on Sione's face said, "Oh my God! He's still here."

I said, "For those of you who kept me, thank you very much. For those who didn't, may you get struck down and die."

Helen glared at me and said, "Now you know why we wanted to vote your ass outta here, right?"

Michael was furious. He felt that Filipe and Sione had stabbed me in the back by saying I'd be "fine" before voting me off. I confronted Filipe.

"You know you wanted me to believe that I had your vote," I said. "That's the truth. No hard feelings. It is what it is, but that's the truth. And if you tell me it's not the truth, then you're lying to me."

Filipe said his Tongan culture had taught him to respect his elders, so he held back his anger.

After this, the show dramatized my Godfather reputation in the house by playing the film's theme music and using Tara's comment about the horse head. They even showed me getting a spa treatment in a robe with cucumbers over my eyes. It was hilarious.

But when Kristin scored below the yellow line with Helen, it really got ugly.

Kristin knew, because of our friendship and the pact I'd made with her mom during the eleventh week, that I would never write her name on that card during an elimination. But she— who had set the record for the first woman in the history of *The Biggest Loser* to lose 100 pounds at the ranch—believed that Michael perceived her as a threat.

She asked me to convince him to vote for her to stay.

"Let me talk to Mike," I told her. "If I can fix it, I will. I love you."

Next, viewers saw the outside of an upstairs window as I whispered to Mike. Our dialogue was printed at the bottom of the screen: "If you guys vote to keep Helen and Filipe and I vote to keep Kristin, Kristin still goes home. She's your biggest threat. Just make sure Tara's on the same page as you."

"Is it okay with you if I do that?" Mike whispered.

"Yeah."

"That's what I want to make sure," Mike answered.

That night, Michael said, during an outdoor interview, "I have the ability to take out the one person who's standing in my way. Can I actually pull the trigger on somebody I love and send them home to make way for me?"

I voted for Helen to leave. The vote was three for Kristin, three for Helen.

Michael voted for Kristin to leave.

She accused him of taking the easy way out to win.

Bob was upset because Kristin had a good chance of winning. He also felt that I was lying about not influencing Michael's decision. I felt terrible that Kristin went home, but the bottom line was that I was there to help Michael.

BECKY
I Hated the Godfather Episode

At our weekly viewing party in our family room, our friends thought it so, so funny that the show was playing *The Godfather* music, because that's their nickname for Ron. He loves to control everything, so it was no surprise when his personality influenced the show.

"Let's rewind it and watch again!" our friends said.

"No, we're not watching it again," I answered.

I hated, hated, hated that portrayal of my husband.

For one, I don't like confrontation with anybody. I didn't like seeing Ron being manipulative, whether it was real or not. Perception is reality, so what America sees on the show is what America believes happened—regardless of what footage ended up on the cutting room floor.

I was sorry to see Kristin leave. I really liked her. But if it came down to her or Michael winning, of course I would vote for my son. I was happy that she'd lost so much weight, and since this was the sixteenth week, the season was almost over.

So in the end, she won too.

Throughout the season, it was obvious to me that Ron was working his magic on the cast. Even though our friends also call him the Godfather, Ron is never outright mean or threatening to anyone. He has a way of being such a nice guy when he's controlling things that people don't realize what's hit them until it's too late.

But when Dane got voted off the show, I knew Ron was pulling strings somehow. That was the only episode that I watched alone in our bedroom. I thought, "How did you do that, Ron?"

As a viewer, I didn't pay much attention to the drama about alliances. I just wanted Michael and Ron to stay and lose weight.

I was especially proud of Michael when he won a year's worth of groceries from General Mills, and then donated them to another contestant.

"I don't need a year's supply of groceries," Michael told Aubrey in her room. He'd won the challenge by loading enough food crates onto trucks at the Los Angeles Regional Food Bank to feed 1,200 people.

"I'm a college student," Michael told Aubrey. "You have five kids. Will you let me give that to you?"

"Oh, that's so awesome, Mike! Yeah!" Aubrey cried. "Thank you!"

"You're welcome," Michael said. He didn't care that Aubrey was on the Blue Team. His heart was in the right place.

Watching at home, I got teary with pride. Especially when Aubrey said, "I couldn't even stop smiling. That was the sweetest thing that anybody could have ever done."

RON
Point of No Return: Going Below Three Hundred Pounds

It was week sixteen when one of the most amazing moments of my life happened as I stepped on the scale.

I reached the point of no return and knew that I had permanently stepped into a new, healthier, and happier life.

Because I weighed 298 pounds.

Going under three hundred was a major benchmark that I had never been able to reach. Every weight-loss plan I'd tried always failed when I got close to three hundred. Fear would plunge me into an eating frenzy and within months I'd be bigger than ever. Now, standing on the scale on *The Biggest Loser*, I was certain that I had left that self-destructive cycle in the dust as my old life as "fat Ron." I was closer than ever to becoming "thin Ron," and I was ecstatic.

"I'm happy," I said told Alison as I remained on the scale. I hadn't been this light since I was thirteen or fourteen years old. "I'm thrilled to death. It's almost unbelievable. But I did it."

Michael ran up and hugged me.

"You did it!" he exclaimed.

I was amazed. I had set a goal to get below three hundred by the finale, but it was only week sixteen.

I cast a grateful look at Bob Harper as he stood with the other contestants. He was making this happen for me. In the gym and in the pool, he knew exactly how I should work out, despite my disabilities. In the kitchen, it was drilled into us to weigh and measure our food and count calories. It became easy to eyeball five ounces of turkey, chop in onions and green peppers, then sizzle up a flavorful, low-fat turkey burger.

Interestingly, I had to learn to eat enough. At one point, my weight plateaued. Bob told me to eat more carbohydrates—half a yam with lunch. Bingo! The pounds started dropping again. He doled out information about nutrition when we needed it, like making sure we ate enough protein with every meal or snack, because protein stokes the metabolism and helps build muscle.

Thanks to Bob, all the information I'd been taught since childhood—and much more—was "clicking." Why it took almost fifty years, I don't know. I'm just grateful that it finally did.

"Being on the Biggest Loser Ranch for me is like the fountain of youth," I said, after Dr. Huizenga told me I no longer needed fourteen pills a day or insulin shots. I was down to one pill every day because losing weight had subdued the diabetes, high blood pressure, and cholesterol.

This time my fear of hitting the three hundred mark was somewhat anticlimactic. I had such good momentum going that that moment sort of came and went. No one was more surprised than me. In the past, fear would cause me to pack on the pounds again and retreat safely into being the "big guy" I'd always been. But this time was different. I told myself, "Okay, I'm past this psychological thing." From then on, I knew I could reach and maintain a normal weight.

During another powerful "lightbulb moment," I understood another thing I'd been hearing my entire life: "Where faith dwells, fear cannot." My faith was carrying me to an amazing place, and I was no longer afraid.

Mike
Point of No Return: Shopping for the Makeover Show

I went to California in size 56 pants. Three months and 110 pounds later, I was home in Michigan, trying on small, cool-looking, trendy jeans in normal sizes at Kohl's. At that moment, while shopping, it hit me that my body had changed dramatically.

I felt like a new person. Confidence tingled through me as I thought, "I don't have to be that obese, miserable guy anymore."

The new clothes symbolized a whole new world of opportunities. This feeling was even more intense when we shopped at Macy's for the show's makeover episode featuring Tim Gunn from the TV show *Project Runway*.

I had lost 140 pounds at that point. Looking at the new Michael Morelli in the three-way mirrors cemented my resolve. I was at the point of no return. I thought, "This is the new me. Forever."

We'd thought we were shopping for outfits to attend a Hollywood movie premiere. But we were really getting ready for the makeover episode. It's a tradition, during every season of *The Biggest Loser*, to devote a whole show to giving makeovers to the contestants who remain. They show video of us when we first started at the ranch and contrast those images with how we look now. They also invite loved ones to join the celebration. Mom and Max flew out to Los Angeles; I was so excited for them to see me and Dad for the first time in months.

To make it even more dramatic, Dad and me and the other contestants would appear at the top of a gilded, red-carpeted staircase while our loved ones waited in shock and awe at the foot of the stairs.

It was so awesome to see my mom's ecstatic face as I stood up there. It was like this moment embodied the best-case scenario for all those times she had tried to help me go on a diet and all those times she suggested I eat something healthier. I had done it and was looking and feeling better than I ever imagined. Stylists had cut my hair, and I wore a dark suit with a turquoise sweater vest.

"Michael looks like a movie star to me," Mom said, standing with Dad and Max. It was phenomenal that we were all sharing this thrilling moment.

I also loved the way Mom was looking at Dad. I can't tell you how many times, when we were fat, she would look disgusted as he brought home pizza for me and Max. Now she looked like she was falling in love with him all over again. She had never seen him clean shaven; the stylists had cut off his beard to symbolize that he was a new man.

Sadly, Max wasn't.

"Why are you crying, Max?"

"I'm the big one," he sobbed.

"Max, it doesn't mean you don't fit into the family," Mom said.

"I feel left out because I'm so big," Max said. "I haven't really, like, done anything about it."

He sat at the foot of the stairs, crying. I tried to comfort him by saying, "Dad and I are coming back, and we're going to get you like this too."

"You're going to be able to do it," Mom said.

When our parents stepped away, I told Max, "I understand how you're feeling. I was there. You feel helpless, right?"

"I just turned seventeen," Max said.

"Just breathe."

"I'm bigger than you were," he said.

"It's not like you're stuck like that," I said. "That's one thing everyone's learned from being here. You have the ability to change, no matter what your situation."

Max cried, "Whenever I see you, I want to be like you." He sniffled. "I want to be seen as normal."

This was one of the most bittersweet moments during my time on the show. I was thrilled with my accomplishment but devastated that Max was hurting.

"We both tried losing weight before at home," I said. "It's hard! Fifteen weeks ago, I thought it was impossible to make this big of a change. I didn't think I would lose this much weight."

I tried to think forward to a moment when I'd be congratulating Max for shrinking to half his size or less.

"You're gonna be amazing," I assured him.

Mike
The Marathon Was Amazing

It was dark on the beach. Seagulls screeched overhead as waves crashed on the sand. Fog rolled in off the ocean.

And I was worried sick about Dad.

He'd been walking for more than thirteen hours through California farmland, mountains, and hiking trails. Now, as I stood on the sand in the chilly night air, I feared his body couldn't take the final trek along the Pacific Coast Highway, which would lead him here.

Bob had warned him not to walk 26.2 miles for the final challenge: a marathon.

But Dad was determined.

"I'm going to do this marathon to show you, Mike and Max, that I'll do anything to right the wrongs of my past," Dad had told us.

"You don't have to, Dad—"

"Yes, I do."

So here I was, waiting and worrying at the finish line. Earlier today Max had flown out to California to join us for part of the marathon, and we had walked part of the marathon together. After flying out to join us, he'd been a real trooper, trudging up hills and highways despite his feet hurting under the weight of his four hundred pounds.

But it was rough. Even I hadn't been able to run the marathon, though I had been training for it. They had sent us home for four weeks just before the marathon and the finale back in California. Being at home threatened to bring my dream to a screeching halt, because I got injured while training in South Lyon. I was running when suddenly it felt like I'd been stabbed in the hip. It was excruciating. My parents took me to the hospital, where doctors said I would not be able to run 26.2 miles.

But I refused to let that stop me. So when I returned to California, I walked the marathon in eight hours, fifty-seven minutes, and six seconds.

But worry about Dad overshadowed my accomplishment as I waited with the other Final Four contestants: Tara, who'd won the marathon, and Helen, who came in second.

"Where is he?" I asked, wishing Mom could have joined us. She had also wondered how Dad would finish a marathon when he couldn't even do a half marathon in December.

Would Dad end up in a wheelchair after this? Would he get chest pains again?

I had no idea that earlier in the day Dad had been shaking uncontrollably, his hands were cold due to poor circulation, his knees were spasming painfully, his blood sugar dropped, and his blood pressure spiked to 202/90!

Dr. H had examined him at the sixteen-mile roadside hydration station, under a tent shielding him from the late afternoon sun.

I would have told Dad to stop trying to play Superman if I had known what was happening to him. He had nothing to prove to me, Max, Bob, or America. He and I had already accomplished so much. During the fifteenth week, I broke a record for the most weight lost (118 pounds!) on the show in *Biggest Loser* history. During week seventeen, Dad and I had surpassed our goal by losing 305 pounds together. Lighter than he'd been in forty years, he'd made it to the Final Four.

Now all I could do was look up to the road where Dad—I hoped—would appear. I'd joined him briefly at mile twenty-one, along with Bob, who was astounded that Dad was still trudging along.

"I didn't say you couldn't do it," Bob exclaimed. "I said you shouldn't do it!"

It was amazing to see winners from five previous seasons walking alongside my dad, cheering him on.

Like me, Tara, and Helen, Dad had a motorcade that included a police car, a minivan full of supplies like water, an ambulance, and a vehicle carrying the camera crew and equipment. A flatbed truck with huge lights was also on hand to film nighttime scenes. This drew tons of attention along the Pacific Coast Highway, a two-lane road with rugged hills and mountains on one side and the beach and ocean on the other.

The caravan around Dad attracted campers from the beach to line the road and cheer, as they had for me, Helen, and Tara. Bob and Jillian also drew tons of cheers.

Another highlight was when winners from previous seasons showed up just as I needed encouragement the most.

But now that I had returned to the finish line on the beach to wait for Dad, I kept looking up at "The Biggest Loser Marathon" finish line. A brown plastic ribbon stretched between the poles and the giant red electronic numbers at the top read 13:10:08, then 13:11:04.

Suddenly the dark, misty sky and road above the beach glowed with silver light. It reminded me of that scene in the movie *Close Encounters of the Third Kind* when spaceship lights illuminate the night sky. Flashing red lights on police cars made it even more dramatic.

Hundreds of people cheered. The caravan was huge; it looked like all the vehicles that had accompanied me, Helen, and Tara were also ushering Dad to the finish line. The round light on the film truck felt as bright as the sun.

Suddenly, Dad's silhouette appeared.

"Thank you, God!" I raised my hands over my face in a prayer position as tears filled my bloodshot eyes. My heart pounded with emotion.

It was like a supernatural vision as Dad—using a cane—stepped onto the sandy path down to the beach. Max was beside him, along with previous winners.

I thought I would just break down and sob as Dad got closer to the finish line. Finally, he raised his cane and whacked down the ribbon. He walked through at 13:15:19 and fell into the biggest embrace with me and Max.

"I love you guys!" Dad exclaimed.

"Good job, Dad!" I sobbed into his shoulder as we hugged for a full minute. "Oh my God!"

People around us cheered, clapped, and cried.

It was one of the most amazing moments of my life, and by far my favorite scene from the entire season. Mom agreed. Friends and complete strangers say they've watched that scene over and over, and they cry every time.

My dad was the ultimate underdog, and he accomplished an amazing feat that most normal-weight people could never do. Fat people don't finish marathons. Nor do people with injured knees. But my dad did. He changed his body, he changed his mind, and he did it for us.

We had one more weigh-in, but it didn't matter. This experience with my dad made my whole family the biggest winners of all.

RON
The Finale Is Just the Beginning

Of course the final weigh-in had a twist: the Final Four contestants didn't get to vote one person off to determine the Final Three contestants. It was up to America to decide which member of the father-and-son team would go to the finale with a chance at becoming the Biggest Loser.

We were the only team from the beginning that was still intact.

"I'm just begging America to vote for my son to be part of the Final Three," I said when it was time to state our case for the viewers to vote by calling in or logging onto the show's Web site.

"I've accomplished every single thing I've wanted to in this competition," Michael told America before the vote. "I've lost 174 pounds. It's just been a privilege being here. If you want to put me in the finale, that's amazing. If you want to put my dad in the finale, that's great too. He deserves it. I love him."

The finale aired live; Becky and Max flew out to Los Angeles to sit in the audience and cheer us on. For Michael and me, it was amazing to be reunited with the twenty other contestants from the beginning of the show. All the drama from those final weeks with Kristin, Sione, and Filipe was replaced with excitement about reuniting and cheering everyone's progress. We'd spent 179 days at the ranch, losing more than 1,400 pounds together. What a bonding experience!

One of the best parts of the finale was bursting through giant "before" pictures of ourselves that were taken when we first came to the ranch. When we'd first talked about auditioning, I remembered how we always took "before" and "after" pictures by the column in our kitchen at the start of our dieting attempts. Now we were celebrating the most phenomenal "after" photos— on live TV!

Michael ripped through the image of his old, obese self—now wearing superslim jeans with a form-fitting blue striped shirt and loafers. As he hugged Alison in her turquoise dress, Becky and Max cheered wildly in the audience.

"This is really crazy!" Michael exclaimed. Live television, as opposed to being filmed by cameras whose footage would be edited for the show, was nerve-racking.

"My dad was my biggest support," Michael said. "Even while we were home, he made sure I did well the entire time."

Alison said, "I think it's time to see how the *Biggest Loser* lifestyle worked for him. Here's Ron!"

I burst through my giant "before" picture. Standing under the bright stage lights beside Michael, I felt like a million bucks in my slim brown suit.

"We both won," I said.

The auditorium exploded with cheers.

"Both of you look amazing," Alison said.

Then came America's choice for the Final Three. Thanks to votes from millions of viewers, Michael made it! Our dream for him to make it to the Final Four had come true. And he looked better than I ever could have imagined. The adrenaline rush of being on stage during a live TV broadcast from Los Angeles felt surreal. I tried to hold on to every second because it felt like it was moving so fast—I'd blink, and it would all be one of the sweetest memories of my life.

Plus, I was very excited and hopeful that I could still become the "at-home" winner for the $100,000 prize. Amazingly, the "oldest contestant," Jerry, won with a total weight loss of 47.97 percent, beating my total of 44.65 percent.

My final weight was 238.

I had lost 192 pounds!

When Michael stepped on the scale, he'd lost a whopping 207 pounds. At 181 pounds, his total weight loss was 53.35 percent.

But Helen dropped 140 pounds, from 257 to 117, with a total loss of 54.47 percent.

Michael lost the title by 1.12 percent.

My heart ached for him because I knew he wanted that title so badly. He had worked so hard! He didn't let his face show it while he stood on stage on live television, but to say he was devastated would be an understatement.

It was such a bittersweet moment. Michael and I had made it to the finale. We were literally half the men we'd been at the start of the show. Yet it could have been even sweeter if I'd won the at-home prize and he became the Biggest Loser. But there wasn't time for regret or disappointment.

Because Michael and I were the biggest winners, with new bodies, new knowledge, new commitments to staying slim. We and the other contestants hugged. Confetti fell from the ceiling. And the audience was going wild.

The Biggest Loser had saved our lives and blessed us with brand-new ones. No money or title could top the miracle of *that*.

During the finale, I couldn't even express my happiness for Dad and Michael. They looked amazing. But as I sat in the audience, cheering beside Mom, nobody knew how torn up I was inside. And it wasn't because I was the only fat one in the family or that my brother was now half my size.

There's more to the story.

I had auditioned for season eight of *The Biggest Loser*. The producers wanted me. We'd done everything required to get on the show: making the video, taking the physical, adjusting my schedule for the end of my junior year. The producers had even told me to pack my bags for five months because after the finale I'd be going to the ranch.

I fantasized about buying normal-size jeans, going on a date with a girl, and just getting comfortably into my car.

But during the finale, the commercial for season eight aired without me. And I thought, "I'll never lose weight."

AN AMAZING OPPORTUNITY APPEARS

Backstage, the owners of the Biggest Loser Resort at Fitness Ridge in Utah approached me and said, "Max, we have a fitness resort and spa, and we want you to come and stay there for the summer. On us."

I was really happy, but Utah seemed so far from my family and friends. Michael and Dad had each other for support at the ranch. I would be alone. Could I do it?

"Max, this is your chance!" Mom gushed.

"We told you it would happen for you too," Dad encouraged.

"You'll be amazing," Michael said.

He was right. Going there was the best decision of my life. I had my own room and ate buffet-style meals in the big, southwestern-style cafeteria. I was pretty amazed that they served low-calorie foods that tasted so good.

Here's the regimen I followed every day.

I'd get up, hike four to eight miles on the mountain trails, then come back for breakfast—usually bran muffins or French toast.

Then I'd go to open gym or a lecture. I also took yoga and exercise classes in the pool and did circuit training in the gym.

Next I'd have lunch. My favorite was shepherd's pie, which they made from scratch. Other times I'd have a sandwich or lettuce wraps. I always hit the salad bar and had fruit for dessert.

In the afternoon, they offered open gym and classes in things like kickboxing or how to lift weights. We also attended lectures by nutritionists, who explained how eating affects your emotions. I realized I was moody in high school because I was eating so much junk. They also had cooking demonstrations and discussions on topics like "intuitive eating," which taught me how to eat only when I was physically hungry instead of when I was bored or lonely.

Nutrition classes taught me to count calories, read labels, estimate normal portions, and not be distracted by TV while eating. I could have learned about calories and fat grams from Mom, at home in our own kitchen, but I had refused to listen.

I also talked with therapists about why I ate. I found it pointless to blame anyone or dwell on the past. I just wanted to improve my future. The whole idea of therapy felt like a waste of time. I wanted to leave my past in the past and spend my energy on making a better future—by losing weight.

For dinner, my favorite meals were turkey burgers and salmon, plus salad and fruit.

The rest of the time, I took long walks with groups in the mountains around the resort or exercised in the gyms. It was so cool to notice progress, like when it was easier to hike up a hill and I didn't get out of breath.

Sometimes I got really tired or feared it would take forever to drop half my weight.

"Just keep going, Max," Dad would say when I called. "There'll be days when you don't want to get out of bed. Just do it." Mom and Michael encouraged me too.

But I felt like I was living in their shadow.

"Oh, you're Mike's brother," starry-eyed men and women would say when they arrived at Fitness Ridge.

Before, I felt like girls and guys couldn't see past my weight to give me a chance at friendship. They couldn't see that there's generally a lot more to overweight people than meets the eye. Now, when people saw me only as Mike's brother, I had the same shallow feeling, like they didn't care specifically about me.

It was hard enough to be far away from home, adjusting to a

new diet and an exhausting exercise routine. Facing my obesity was really tough. I couldn't bury my feelings in food, so they surged up.

"Why am I doing this?" I'd sometimes wonder. "Why am I still here? What's going on at home? What do I want to do after this?" I was really irritable because I missed my friends. We talked, texted, and e-mailed, but I still felt out of the loop. I just wanted to go home and enjoy my summer. But I was still fat.

That's when I'd remind myself that "I need to be here!"

My little fits were stupid because I was so glad to be losing weight. And I am so grateful to the owners of Fitness Ridge for giving me this awesome experience. A typical three month-stay would have cost more than $21,000.

Still, it really pissed me off when people compared me to my brother. I felt like everyone expected me to be like him and Dad, and not my own person. Sometimes people would ask me questions about my dad and brother, as if I were a walking, talking celebrity tabloid magazine. I'd think, "I'm not here to keep you entertained," and I'd retreat to the gym to work off my bad mood. I hated when people acted like they knew us really well, but they didn't.

The same thing happened on Facebook. I love all the people who've supported me. I actually have four thousand "friends." But I ignore people who friend me just to ask about Dad and Michael.

"You look amazing!" Michael said when I came home in August. More than a hundred pounds lighter, I felt as confident as when I was a nine-year-old Little League baseball star.

Finally I was becoming the person I wanted to be. And it was the best feeling ever. But I still needed to lose a hundred more pounds. And coming home for my senior year in high school—and the temptation of all my bad habits from the past—made me terrified that I'd pack the pounds back on.

CHAPTER 12

MIKE

Fighting Fat and Getting Fit in College

The first time I came to college, I weighed 397 pounds—my heaviest ever. My belly was so big that I could hardly climb into the sleeping loft in my dorm room.

Fast-forward to August 2009, when I returned to MSU to restart my freshman year.

At 225 pounds, I was a new man.

Since leaving the ranch, I had become a certified personal trainer. But it was tough being home all summer amid constant temptation. I had gained forty-four pounds since the finale.

The following summer, 2010, was fortunately a different story. I actually lost weight, getting down to 215 pounds. I've been working hard to build muscle and tone my body into its best shape ever, and I now feel nothing short of amazing.

Even more amazing was running the Morelli Health and Fitness Camp in our hometown. It was the best experience for me and my dad to share our *Biggest Loser* journey and knowledge to help nine overweight kids learn how to eat healthy meals and lose weight. They spent nine hours a day, five days a week, with us for most of the summer. We'd start in a home economics room at a local school, where we taught them how to cook scrambled egg whites and turkey bacon for breakfast or chicken with vegetables for lunch.

The kids were so used to eating fast food that they were hesitant to try something new and healthy. Just like Max and I once thought, our campers believed that anything healthy had to taste bad. It was so cool to watch them actually enjoy the healthy food they cooked with no oil.

Anytime Fitness, our local gym, let them work out for free; it was awesome to watch the kids' excitement grow as they became faster and stronger.

I pushed one boy especially hard because, at age thirteen, he was like a mini version of me at that age. When I first saw him, I just stared because I couldn't believe the similarity. That put me on a mission to spare him from growing into the four-hundred-pound teenager I once was. I can't even express the joy of watching the excitement in his eyes as I got him to run at eleven miles an hour on the treadmill. He was beaming with accomplishment. By the end of the summer, he'd lost thirty-five pounds!

That is the gift I am now sharing with others, thanks to my amazing transformation on *The Biggest Loser*.

Now, back at college, I'm still working on building muscle and trimming fat. During the fall of my freshman year, I devised a food-and-fitness routine that can help any college student, whether living in a dormitory or an off-campus apartment. If you take a look at my typical daily routine during my freshman and sophomore years, you'll see how I managed to beat obesity at college, and you can too.

During my freshman year, I lived in a dormitory and shared a room with my best friend from first grade. Now I live in an off-campus apartment. In both places, my morning routine has remained the same: The first thing I do is weigh myself. This motivates me to stick to my regimen all day, so the next morning's weigh-in flashes a number that makes me feel good. If I blow it, the scale will show it. Gaining weight freaks me out, because I never want to look and feel as horrible as I did before the show.

Next, after I put on normal-size jeans and get dressed, I glance at superfit guys in *Men's Health, Men's Fitness*, and *Muscle and Fitness*. Stacks of magazines cover my desk and bookshelves. I love the articles about workouts and healthy eating; they keep me disciplined.

For me, being disciplined means eating 1,800 calories a day and exercising every day except Sunday. I'm always pushing toward the next goal. Losing 207 pounds on *The Biggest Loser* and setting a record for the most weight lost on the show proved to me that I can achieve anything. But it also set my standards very high, and I stay in a constant state of striving to challenge myself. Once you achieve your best, like I did at the ranch, mediocrity feels like failure.

"I have really changed my life," I said during the finale. "When I first started this journey, I hated myself. I felt that I was disgusting. Now I know that I can do anything I set my mind to. I embarked on this journey when I was only eighteen years old. Now I have my entire life in front of me. There's nothing that's going to stop me now."

I still feel that way.

But when I give motivational talks about losing weight, or when people on campus ask me how to slim down, I don't sugar-coat the truth.

The bottom line is that you have to channel your self-hatred and disgust into mental and physical energy to change your body. Most people will never get a *Biggest Loser* moment.

In real life, it's all on you. Every day, I *make* myself work out. I *make* myself eat healthily. I *force* myself to resist temptation.

So, if you want to lose weight, you have to hate yourself

enough to want to change, but not hate yourself so much that you spiral into despair.

And even if you saw me lose twenty-two pounds during my first week on the show, it's not realistic or safe for the average person to lose that much weight at home.

You have to take pleasure in little victories. Instead of saying, "Oh, man, I lost only two pounds this week," say enthusiastically, "I lost two pounds this week! That's a great step toward a better me."

A lot of people won't admit that hating yourself plays a part in this transition. But on some level, every heavy person feels it. And hating yourself is the best catalyst to one day saying, "I love myself!" You want to look in the mirror and love the way you look. You want to go shopping for clothes and get skinny jeans or a form-fitting shirt and smile at yourself in the mirror.

Most importantly, you want to feel in control of food, not like food is controlling you.

You have to toughen your mind. Because, believe me, temptation is always there. Twenty-four hours a day, seven days a week. The foodaholic beast within me never rests.

On campus slipping back into old habits is as easy as dialing the phone to order a pizza or stepping into the entrée line in the cafeteria for a cheeseburger and fries, with a stop at the dessert station for chocolate chip cookies. Or chowing down on late-night snacks with my roommates.

I *never* do that. But the temptation is there, and it's even worse on football Saturdays. Since I could see the nearby stadium from my dorm room, I could also smell the meat grilling at tailgate parties in every parking lot for as far as I could see. The parties are a foodaholic's paradise, serving doughnuts, chili dogs, chips, and practically every fattening food you can imagine.

During my freshman year, the show visited me on a football

Saturday for a "where are they now?" segment that aired during Thanksgiving week 2009. Jillian and a camera crew joined me and my family at a huge tailgate party where everyone was chowing down on fattening fare. Not me. I think I ate an apple, and I had already hit the gym that morning.

CALORIES IN, CALORIES OUT ON CAMPUS

So what do I eat on a typical day?

In the morning, when I lived in the dorm, I would head down to the cafeteria—"the caf" as we called it—to meet about five friends. We always sat at the same table, under a bright solarium overlooking trees, grass, and another modular red-brick dormitory where I work out.

In the cafeteria, I acted like I was wearing blinders, ignoring the food that other students were eating, like heaping mounds of scrambled eggs, Cocoa Puffs, and buttered French toast drizzled with maple syrup. I ate the same breakfast every day: three hard-boiled eggs, half a glass of milk, Kashi GoLean cereal (when they had it), and an apple. I'm not a breakfast person, but I force myself to eat because it jump-starts my metabolism for the day.

In my apartment, I eat oatmeal prepared with milk. It's much easier to regulate my food when I do my own grocery shopping and make sure that certain items, such as cookies, are not in the house.

After breakfast, I dash off to class. The MSU campus is huge, but most of my freshman classes were no more than a ten-minute walk from the dorm. As a sophomore, I still walk a lot. I love school and always have. After the show, I changed my premed major to kinesiology. I'm planning to attend medical school to study sports medicine, then become a team doctor for an NFL team.

During my freshman year, I took fifteen credits per semester, with classes such as: Introduction to Athletic Training, Clinical Observation of Athletic Training, Health and Nutrition, First Aid, Yoga, and Men in America (lots of writing). Since exercise and eating healthily are a huge part of my day, it's cool that I got to study—and still do—my favorite subjects in class. I liked Fridays best, when I actually got to apply tape to athletes' ankles in the football training center.

I still get to do that this year, in addition to classes such as Healthy Lifestyle and Pathology of Sports Injury.

After class I return to my apartment and have a tuna sandwich on wheat bread. (I go through phases where I eat the same foods, such as a Greek salad topped with grilled chicken.) If I'm still hungry, I'll have some cottage cheese and an apple. I love being able to prepare my own food in the healthiest way possible.

As I mentioned, when I lived in the dorm I ate lunch in the cafeteria. Since I had the "silver meal plan," I had unlimited swipes on my meal card. For lunch, I would head to the salad bar, over which hung a "Well-Being" sign. I would build a Greek salad with tuna and vinaigrette dressing, plus an apple for dessert. Sometimes I made a whole-wheat wrap with tuna, lettuce, tomato, mustard, and light mayonnaise. The salad bar also had a Mediterranean section, where I often got a scoop of one of my favorite foods: hummus.

When other students ask me how to make healthy eating choices in the cafeteria, here's what I say:

- *Check your options.* Don't just get in the entrée line and take whatever they give you. Walk around and look at everything first: the salad bar, the fresh fruit baskets, healthy cereals, other protein options like yogurt, cottage cheese, hard-boiled eggs, and tuna. You can build a healthier meal this way.

- *Go for a plate of colors.* Colorful vegetables and fruit will fill you up with lots of vitamins and few calories.

- *Have nature's candy for dessert.* Fresh fruit. It's sweet, it's delicious, and you won't feel guilty.

- *Have a schedule.* If the cafeteria is the hang-out spot for your friends, and you find yourself there six times a day, you'll end up snacking while chatting. Instead go to the cafeteria only for breakfast, lunch, and dinner.

- *Don't be too strict.* Follow the motto "everything in moderation." Restricting yourself with off-limit foods will only make you want them more.

- *Calories in, calories out.* This is obvious, but you have to count the number of calories you're taking in, both to make sure you're eating the right amount and to know how much exercise you need to do to lose weight. Online calorie counters can calculate how many calories your body needs in a day, depending on your age, height, weight, and gender. And you'll have to do some basic research about how many calories different foods typically have, so you can make smart decisions in the cafeteria. Then make a food plan accordingly.

- *Set your own rules.* I've stopped eating meat in the cafeteria as a way to cut calories. Sometimes, for example, they serve a taco salad. I initially thought, "It's just a salad." But I had to get real with myself. It's a salad in a fried tortilla shell stuffed with ground beef, cheese, and sour cream. That adds up to a lot of calories. Same with a beef chimichanga, which I love. I realized that it's not only fried in a flour tortilla but it's full of high-calorie beef and surrounded by cheese and sour cream.

After lunch, I head to classes. Then I return to my apartment (or dorm room during freshman year), change into shorts and a T-shirt, and go to the gym. I can't sit down or get comfortable; I have to keep moving so I don't get lazy and skip my workout.

It takes a minute to get my head in the right place for a good workout. I need to be really mad to lift weights and give it my all. So I listen to my iPod and play angry, aggressive songs. My music playlist is usually "Lose Yourself" and "'Till I Collapse" by Eminem, "Many Men" by 50 cent, "To Be Loved" by Papa Roach, "Party and Bullshit" by Biggie Smalls, "Moment of Clarity" by Jay-Z, "I Stand Alone" by Godsmack, "Cult of Personality" by Living Colour, "Remember the Name" by Fort Minor, and "A Country Boy Can Survive" by Hank Williams Jr.

Then I either think about something that pissed me off that day or I imagine someone being mean to my brother. That pushes me into an adrenaline-fueled rage that turbocharges my body to pump iron.

If I'm annoyed, I think, "I gotta take a run," or "I need to go hit the punching bag in the gym."

I love sharing my knowledge by training two students on campus. I hone my grueling workouts—distilled from fitness magazines and everything I learned from Bob and Jillian—into customized workouts for them. My clients are losing weight and getting toned. It's no wonder, since I have them doing "the leg matrix." That's thirty-six lunges, thirty-six squats, thirty-six jumping lunges, thirty-six jumping squats—all in a row, twice. It's painful. But it shows results.

Body weight exercises like these are my favorite; I do a lot of them, along with free weight work, bench presses, the squat rack, the lat pull-down machine, and sit-ups on the incline bench.

I'm doing a lot of abdominal work, striving for a six-pack, thanks to skin surgery. On December 22, 2009, I had an operation to remove six and a half pounds of loose skin from my abdomen. When my giant belly disappeared, deflated skin remained. Now I have an upside-down, red, T-shaped scar from my breastbone to my groin, and around my hips. Unlike Dad, I had no external stitches. They "glued" the incision with stitches that dissolved. I had drainage tubes for a while, until the scar healed. It was gross but worth it, because I feel so much better with skin that fits my new body.

Since the scar is not stretchy like normal skin, I have to be careful when working out. Sometimes when I'm bench-pressing, I'll feel something weird and wonder, "Did I just explode something in my gut?" I'm also careful, during yoga, not to twist a certain way to aggravate the scar.

I'm cautious with my knee too, because I developed bursitis during the show. If I run too hard or do certain leg exercises on the weight machines, it hurts.

I don't love cardio training, but I try to run outside at least three times a week, even during the winter. I also play defense for intramural soccer once a week, as well as racquetball. Some days I'll take two spinning classes in a row or spend the whole day in the gym if I don't have class.

"You're a beast!" my roommate teases.

After my workout, it's time for dinner. When I lived in the dorm, I ate with five to eight friends in the cafeteria. The meal was pretty much a repeat of lunch: a Greek salad and cooked vegetables, like the veggie medley or roasted asparagus, then fruit for dessert.

I'm a cookie guy, and it was pure torment at lunch and din-ner to pass the dessert cart on the way to the cafeteria exit. It was loaded with giant cookies, cake, and brownies.

Fortunately, I have a close-knit group of friends who put me in check when my discipline slips. If I sat down in the caf with a beef chimichanga on my tray, they'd say, "Mike, really?"

And I'd say no and get rid of it.

Those temptations aren't a problem in my apartment, because I just don't buy that junk. Dinner is usually something like tuna, cooked green beans that I buy frozen, cottage cheese and almonds, and an apple.

I stay pretty busy with homework, exercise, parties, and sports, so I avoid any after-dinner temptation to snack.

But living in the dorm—that was torturous. The hardest part of the day was evening, because every night someone was order-ing Jimmy John's sandwiches or pizza or fried cheese sticks. And get this: there's a place called Insomnia Cookies that's open from 4:00 p.m. until 4:00 a.m. You call and order your favorite kind of cookies; then they make them fresh and deliver them to the dorm. Warm! That is a food addict's dream and nightmare all rolled into one phone call! My roommate ordered them all the time; those double chocolate chunk cookies looked so good. But I haven't tried them. I don't want to set off the foodaholic who would probably put Insomnia Cookies on speed dial.

When temptation struck, I talked myself through it. "Am I hungry? No. How will I feel after I eat it? Bad. Are a few minutes of pleasure worth hours and days of guilt? No."

If I did have a cookie in the cafeteria, it was okay. It was just one cookie, not eight, like I used to eat. Keeping everything in moderation is the key to my success.

Even though I've had huge success losing weight and keep-ing it off, I'm still intimidated by certain things. Like the weight room in the Intramural Sports Building. It's full of huge guys who've been lifting weights for years. I never even go in there.

What about alcohol? MSU knows how to throw a party, but drinking down hundreds of calories in beer or sugary mixed drinks is a diet disaster.

So when I go to parties, I fill a flask with sugar-free Hawaiian punch. I blend right in with all the people around me who are getting drunk. If someone offers me a shot, I give it to someone else.

Now that I'm a normal-weight guy, I feel more confident when talking to people. During my freshman year, I was still getting comfortable with the new me. But now, during my sophomore year, I feel like I've really grown into the new Mike. People tell me all the time that I look and seem much happier. I am. I'm more relaxed and more at peace with myself. I feel in control of what goes into my body. I have no need to look back and analyze the past. I'm grateful for all my experiences because that's what brought me to the point where I am now, and I love myself now.

That doesn't mean that it's easy to avoid the temptation of food. I still love to eat. I stick to my strict regimen during the week; then on the weekends I allow myself to indulge in sandwiches from Jimmy John's or I eat chips and dip while watching football. When our family took a seven-day Caribbean cruise in August 2010, I ate what I wanted and was at peace with the fact that I was on vacation and could relax my rules, with the agreement that I would get back on my regimen once I returned to campus. I loved the lobster and enjoyed things like mashed potatoes and gravy, bread with butter, and desserts. I still ate salads and veggies too. This balance is the ultimate way of enjoying life. And I love it!

Back at school, when I'm out with friends, food always comes into the picture. After a party, everybody wants to go out to eat or to order a pizza. Sometimes I'm taunted by fattening food twenty-four hours a day.

But I have many tricks for overcoming temptation.

"Nothing tastes as good as being fit feels," I tell myself, over and over.

I also have two pictures in my wallet: one of me before the show, at nearly 400 pounds, and the other of me weighing 181 at the finale. While I'm looking at these pictures, I think of that scene on the show when Dr. H showed me pictures of my sixty-five-inch belly after I'd already lost a ton of weight.

"I didn't know how huge I was," I told him as I stared in absolute disgust and awe at the picture of my formerly enormous belly. That memory is the ultimate appetite suppressant. Then I look at my "before" and "after" pictures from my wallet and think, "Which is better? Which do I want to be today?"

"After" always wins.

CHAPTER **13** / **MAX**

Fighting Fat and Getting Fit in High School

Kids don't listen to their parents.

Take it from me.

If I had listened to my mom about eating better and being more active, I would never have weighed four hundred pounds.

I was more receptive to learning how to eat well and exercise when I went away to Fitness Ridge.

I was lucky, but it got me thinking that school is the best place for kids to learn how to eat healthy and exercise. That's where we're more open to learning from an outside source. We want to learn because the truth is that a lot of kids are sick of being overweight. But since they're so fat and they lack the tools to change, they're lost.

I think schools should have fun, realistic programs that teach kids about nutrition, healthy foods that taste good, and exercise. Kids also have no concept of the long-term consequences of eating badly and being inactive. We need to learn that we can get sick and die from putting junk into our bodies every day. I think it's great that some schools are changing their lunch menus and removing pop machines.

Meanwhile, I hope my tips can help high school kids fight fat and get fit:

- *Get active!* Those two little words can make a huge impact on a kid's life. Go outside. Toss around a Frisbee with your friends. Take a walk. Don't sit inside and watch TV or play video games. Play volleyball or football. You'll have so much fun that you'll forget you're exercising.

You can also join a gym. I go to the gym every day except Sunday. I do strength training to build muscle, and I do a cardio workout to burn off fat.

- *Take it slow.* You gained weight bite by bite, so you have to lose weight calorie by calorie. Go online or ask your doctor to figure out how many calories you should eat in a day to safely lose weight, and find out what the normal weight for your age and height should be. It's all about the numbers, and, believe me, you will see the difference on the scale. If I can go from over four hundred pounds to under three hundred, then you can do it too.

- *Find a new outlet.* Food can be your best friend if you're stressed. Girls always go to ice cream when they're upset. Guys eat for comfort too. But you have to find a healthier way to blow off steam. Write in a journal. Call a friend. Find a hobby that uses your hands so you can't eat (like working on cars, painting, or building model airplanes).

For me, working out replaced running to food when I'm bored or upset. Eating might make you feel good for a little while, but the guilt and the nausea make you feel worse. Exercise always makes you feel better. Now it's automatic. If something upsets me, I hit the gym.

- *Fast food doesn't have to be fattening.* I won't lie—it's tough watching my buddies chow down on chili cheese fries while I'm eating a Greek salad with grilled chicken. Fortunately, the excitement of finally losing weight makes me not want to eat thousands of calories in one sitting anymore. And now that I've reprogrammed my brain to compute calories, I think about how many hours I'd have to spend in the gym to burn off all that greasy cheese, meat, and fries. It's not worth it.

Fortunately, a lot of fast-food places now have healthy options. Taco Bell has the Fresco menu. Or you can go to Subway and get a healthy sub with 260 calories. You might have to be willing to make adjustments as well. For example, if you go to McDonald's and order the Southwest Salad, you could ask them not to put the tortilla chips on top. And use just a small amount of dressing.

- *Psych yourself out.* I tell myself that I hate grease and hate salt. I tell myself that I just don't like pizza anymore. I tell myself that I don't need to eat a lot. And most of the time, it works. In my mind, I equate junky fast food with feeling and looking horrible. That makes me lose my appetite for junk.

- *Eat what you like.* I live on turkey sandwiches. I use whole wheat bread that has thirty-five calories per slice, and I eat the same sandwich for lunch and dinner. I also like fruit with fat-free whipped cream for breakfast or a protein bar or an 80-calorie cup of yogurt. My mom makes awesome vegetable soup, but I don't like chunks in my soup, so she purees it for me. That's what I like. That's what works. It's really important that you eat what you like so you'll stick with it.

- *Avoid tempting environments.* I had to stop working at McDonald's because being there made it too easy to eat free Double Cheeseburgers.

- *Hang around supportive people.* My best friend since I was seven years old, Colin, always has my back. If we're hanging out and there's a bowl of Doritos or tortilla chips sitting around, he'll put it away. A lot of my friends can tell when I'm tempted, so they remove the temptation, and it makes things easier on me.

- *Don't diet.* If you wake up in the morning and think, "I'm on a diet," you're doomed to failure. It's a lot like when your parents tell you to do something: you don't want to do it. If somebody says, "You can never eat chocolate cake," you'll become obsessed with having chocolate cake. It's just a weird mind game. And "diet" is definitely a four-letter word in that game. So say, "I'm eating healthily today so I'll look and feel better." Say that over and over to convince yourself. And you'll succeed.

After high school graduation, I went back to Fitness Ridge for six weeks, during the summer of 2010.

I feel awesome! I lost another 48 pounds there. When I left, in mid-June, I weighed 326. The routine was pretty much the same as the first time I went, the year before. I'd start the morning with a hike on the mountain trails. I'd eat meals that they prepared in the cafeteria, strictly following a 1,200-calorie-a-day plan. I loved their breakfast muffins, turkey sandwiches, and bell peppers stuffed with eggplant. The rest of the day, I exercised and took classes about nutrition.

When I came home in late July, I weighed 278 pounds. Over the rest of the summer, I dropped more weight. Now I'm 270.

It's amazing how I feel—lighter, more energetic, happier. Like this giant load has literally been lifted from my body. I can do so many more things with my friends, like play Frisbee or volleyball at the sand court in the middle of our town. I'm not dating, but I go out with my friends a lot, and I feel like I'm having way more fun.

The best thing is that I'm much happier and more relaxed. I have a more laid-back outlook, like I'm going to live life day by day and keep going in the best direction for me. I have no reason to sit down and be like, "Where did I go wrong all those years ago?" Back then I was so mad at myself, depressed, sad. I'm a completely different person now. I feel in control of my body and emotions, so I'm not angry or moody as much.

I'm still working on losing more weight. My plan is to return to Fitness Ridge whenever I have a big chunk of free time.

For now, though, I've started classes at Oakland Community College. My focus is accounting and acting. I'm taking five classes, for fifteen credits, in the following subjects: accounting, film, history, algebra, and English. Eventually, I want to transfer to Michigan State (I visit Michael there a lot on weekends) or University of Georgia or UCLA. My goal is to become an actor with accounting as my "plan B."

School keeps me really busy, but I still go to the gym five or six times a week. I'm lucky to still live at home, where Mom and Dad are always giving me support, stocking the kitchen with healthy food, and making sure I stick to my plan. Here's how I maintain my weight right now.

For breakfast, I have scrambled Egg Beaters with turkey bacon. If I don't have time to cook, I grab a protein bar and eat it while driving to school.

For lunch, I eat a turkey sandwich and a low-fat, fruit-flavored yogurt if I'm at home. If I'm near campus, I go to Subway and get a chicken breast sub on wheat, with no dressing and no cheese.

For dinner, I have a turkey roll-up (sliced turkey rolled up in a reduced-calorie wheat tortilla). I should eat more fruits and vegetables. If Mom has made green beans, or cut up fruit like watermelon, cantaloupe, or pineapple, I have a serving of that.

My goal is to get down to the best weight for me—under two hundred pounds—and kick into autopilot with my eating and exercise. That will be the new "normal" for my life, and talking about the old, obese Max will no longer be part of the conversation. I'll be too busy having fun and loving life.

Meanwhile, I hope my tips can help you lose weight and feel better. You're welcome to friend me on Facebook and say, "Hey, Max, it worked! I followed your advice, and I lost weight!"

I'll see you online. Good luck!

CHAPTER 14 / BECKY

Make Health a Family Affair

My greatest regret in life is that I allowed my children to become obese. I will never forgive myself for that.

Now, thankfully, we're all in a much better place, and I wanted to share our experience to help other families avoid our mistakes or undo the damage that's already been done.

First, our family is proof that no one will lose weight until they're truly ready. I was eager to help us get fit by stocking the kitchen with healthy foods and preparing creative, low-calorie meals. But the boys were having more fun with Ron, who did not share my commitment to better eating and exercise.

Second, Ron himself is proof that no magic solution exists. Even gastric bypass surgery didn't ensure that he would keep the weight off. His body was altered, but his mind wasn't ready.

Looking back, I could have taken more control of the boys' future weights by serving healthier meals when they were very small and insisting that they eat more balanced meals. But hindsight is twenty-twenty, so instead of dwelling on the past I have to learn from it and look toward a healthier future. I could consider the "could've" and "should've" ideas all day long, but it won't change the past.

Instead I offer the following tips to help your family beat obesity, just like mine did.

- *Eat dinner together as a family.* This allows the parent who cooks to control the quality and quantities of foods that are prepared and served. This also makes the dinner table a place to bond, enjoy one another, and discuss issues.

When both parents are committed to raising healthy, normal-weight children, they will control their portion sizes and set a good example for the kids.

For us, abandoning the kitchen table was a huge mistake. Like most families with working parents and busy kids, it was so easy to grab a pizza or fast food and eat on the couch while watching TV. Research shows that kids and adults eat more food in front of the television. Being at the table with parents' watchful eyes instills boundaries about when a balanced meal begins and ends.

- *Make eating out an occasional treat, not the norm.* Restaurant portions are huge, and they're often made with extra butter, oil, and salt to enhance flavor. Kids menus are loaded with high-fat favorites like chicken strips, burgers, fries, grilled cheese, mac 'n' cheese, and pizza. Refills on pop can add hundreds of calories to a meal, as can fun appetizers like fried mozzarella sticks or bloomin' onions (that's an entire onion cut almost to the bottom, to form a flowerlike shape; it's dipped in batter, fried, and enjoyed with creamy dip). I won't even talk about the dessert menu!

We became a fat family by eating out, sometimes twice a day. Fast food was always around. The kids didn't drive and had no way to go purchase the crap that came in the bags from the drive-through unless *we* took them there. And we did. Again and again. It makes me very sad to realize how our bad habits became the kids' bad habits.

Have the courage to say no to kids who want the latest toy at a fast-food place. Think in terms of the big picture—how a few hundred extra calories several times a week add up to pounds in months and years.

- *If "food is love" in your home, find a new way to express love.* This isn't easy. On Valentine's Day, I was so tempted to make chocolate chip cookies for Michael, but I didn't because that would sabotage his efforts to avoid his main "trigger food" that could set off a binge, weight gain, and guilt. Instead I scheduled time for us to go to the gym, where he could show me how to lift light weights to strengthen my arm muscles. That was even better than cookies; we spent quality time together, focusing on something that promotes better health for our family.

- *Re-create family traditions for holiday meals.* We are no longer faced with the temptation of huge buffets of fattening food on holidays, because we now plan and prepare our own meals with low-fat, healthy recipes. It seems like everyone uses the holidays as an excuse to eat with wild abandon, only to go on a diet (that usually fails) in January. The result? Five or ten more pounds carried into the New Year. We have taken charge of this seemingly all-American tradition, and it's so liberating to wake up on January first without the dread or guilt of weight gain and dieting.

- *Plan the family's meals in advance and cook a large amount.* It's best to shop and cook on your days off, so that healthy foods are available when you, your spouse, or your kids get hungry throughout the week.

If you don't know how to prepare balanced meals, take a nutrition class or do research online. Every meal should include a lean protein like baked fish or broiled chicken, a salad and/or vegetable, and a small portion of starch like half a baked sweet potato or a half cup of rice. Using small amounts of "healthy fats" like olive oil is important too. Serve fruit for dessert. Keep healthy snacks like fruit and 100-calorie snack packs to satisfy cravings and tide kids over until mealtimes.

We thought we were saving time and energy by eating out. But we paid a terrible price when the boys became obese.

The investment you make in meal planning, shopping, and cooking will pay the best dividend ever: a healthy, normal-weight family.

- *Keep it simple!* We don't make elaborate low-fat recipes. We eat the same simple foods every day. That's what works for us, because we don't have to stop and think about whether we should eat this or that. We know that what's in our refrigerator is healthy and low in calories, and we know that what we eat every day enables us to maintain our weights and feel great.

For example, Ron makes four-ounce patties with ground turkey, black pepper, and onion powder. He freezes them on a cookie sheet, then puts the frozen patties into individual plastic containers. When mealtime comes, he pops one onto the George Foreman Grill, and voilà! He's got a burger.

Our refrigerator's cheese drawer contains several types of low-fat or nonfat cheeses for sandwiches. Our bread box on the counter has all kinds of low-calorie, whole wheat bread and buns. I prefer to spend a little more money to purchase prepackaged things like chicken breasts, low-fat salad dressing, and low-fat yogurts. That gives me automatic portion control and takes the guesswork out of calorie counting.

Our pantry has brown rice, pasta, and yams, all of which we eat in moderation. There's a digital scale sitting on our kitchen island so that we can weigh foods and make sure we're eating appropriate portions.

We prepare foods without adding extra calories. We do not fry or use oil to prepare meats. I use I Can't Believe It's Not Butter spray, which has zero calories. Ron would rather enjoy the taste of real butter or mayonnaise by using a small amount. If there's a nonfat version available, I'll buy it because I don't mind a slight sacrifice in taste and texture to save calories.

- *Don't keep junk food, sweets, or trigger foods in the house.* This is one of my top rules. If the cabinets contain no chips or cookies, and no fried chicken or pizza is in the refrigerator, then no one can eat that stuff. If you or someone in your family has no control around certain foods, don't buy them. And as the parents, you control what you buy at the grocery store. Stop thinking of fattening foods as a treat; they're really the opposite.

Recently, I had a strong craving for ice cream in the evening. But we didn't have any in the house, so I ate watermelon. It was sweet and delicious. The next morning, I felt great because I hadn't eaten all those calories from ice cream. At other times, if I want to indulge my craving, I'll purchase a small, single-serving container of low-fat ice cream. It satisfies me without the guilt.

Michael loves cookies. Max loves chips. Ron loves peanut butter. I know not to keep those things in the house because they will disappear and show up stuck to someone's fat cells the next day. If it's not in the house, we can't eat it. And if we don't buy it, it's not in the house.

- *Make exercise a daily fun activity for everyone.* The whole family can take a walk. Go bike riding together. Go roller-skating. The list of fun activities parents can use to get kids moving is endless.

In our heavier days, Ron and I took the boys to the park. But we'd sit on a bench while they played. Now we take walks together, and I even go to the gym with Michael when he's home from college.

- *Don't scold the kids if they eat junk.* That only makes a child or teen feel worse, which can trigger comfort eating. Make conversations about eating a part of daily life so it's not a big deal. Keep an ongoing dialogue, so that when the kids indulge in burgers and fries one day, they'll be more active and eat lighter and leaner the next day.

This advice was tested in our house recently when Michael had a late-night cookie binge. Rather than question him or scold him, I let the situation take care of itself.

The next day, he ate a Greek salad with chicken breast and spent extra time in the gym. He knew what he needed to do, and he didn't need me to remind him or make him feel worse.

- *Make sure you still have fun; don't let healthy eating ruin your social life.* Ron and I have such a fun social life that Michael teased us one Saturday evening when we stayed home and watched a movie. "Now you're finally acting your age," he said playfully. The comment referred to a costume party we'd attended as Minnie and Mickey Mouse. We play euchre with our large circle of longtime friends on Saturday nights, and we go out for dinner with our friends on Friday evenings. That's when we relax our eating, to enjoy beer, pizza, and other treats that we avoid during the week. Our healthy eating has not hindered our social life; our friends are extremely supportive of our commitment to be a fit family.

- *Be a great role model, and don't lose hope.* During all those years when Ron and the boys were eating bad, and I was sticking to my regimen, I never gave up hope that one day they'd see the light.

I'm proof that you don't need to become a contestant on a TV show like *The Biggest Loser* to get thin and healthy. Even though I had bariatric surgery, it still takes commitment and discipline to keep the weight off.

Here's a look at my regimen:

5:30 a.m. Workout: One hour of cardio and strength training.

Breakfast: Becky's Breakfast Sandwich: a whole grain English muffin filled with Egg Beaters and low-fat cheese.

Morning Snack: A yogurt or high-fiber cereal (dry).

Lunch: A salad with two ounces of lean protein and lots of veggies, and fat-free or light dressing.

Afternoon Snack: A Fiber One Bar or air-popped corn.

Dinner: Three ounces of lean protein with *lots* of veggies and whole grain bread or brown rice.

Evening Snack: Watermelon, popcorn, light ice cream, or fat-free pudding.

It's really important to create a plan that works for you, your tastes, and your schedule.

You can also make a family plan with foods and activities everyone enjoys. The bottom line is making a plan and sticking to it, even when the kids say they'd rather eat pizza while watching TV.

As parents, you have the power to help your kids beat obesity. It's easier to say no to fast food one night than to watch your child grow up into an unhappy, four-hundred-pound teenager risking illness and death.

Take it from us: prevention is your best medicine.

CHAPTER **15** / **RON**

No More Fear, No More
Excuses

When Michael and I flew back to Michigan after *The Biggest Loser* finale in May 2009, we didn't have to ask for seatbelt extenders. We only needed two seats, and our legs were not squeezing against the sides. Nobody gave us dirty looks. And we could actually lower the tray tables and enjoy a Diet Coke.

All because we were four hundred pounds lighter than when we'd flown to California eight months before.

Coming home was the start of a new life for both of us. No one is more shocked than I am to discover a lasting solution to my lifetime struggles as a foodaholic. The beast still lives within me. I may never kill it. The difference now is that I control it; it doesn't control me.

What I learned at the ranch about eating and exercise was so life changing, that now I want to go up to every heavy person I see in public and say something, anything, to help them escape their deadly habits and feel as great as I do.

NO MORE EXCUSES!

Fat was the ultimate excuse to let fear hold me back from living life to the fullest. Every time I got close to three hundred pounds, sheer terror would strike, rouse the beast, and boom! I'd retreat to a fog of food and fat, where I felt too lousy about myself to care anymore.

But something happened at the ranch when I weighed in at 298. Nothing. I just kept going. Because finally I realized that I could do it.

Now I want to help you get rid of the excuses that are holding you back from living a full, healthy, happy life. I've heard them all; they used to come out of my own mouth.

EXCUSE: *I can't lose weight because . . .*
THE TRUTH: Yes, you can! That's exactly how Bob and Jillian responded to us in the gym if we dared utter "I can't." If I could walk a marathon on two bum knees, then you can push past your limits and surprise yourself with what you can do in the gym.

EXCUSE: I'm too old, with too many health problems, to exercise and lose weight.
THE TRUTH: No you're not! People come up to me all the time to ask how they—at age fifty or sixty or seventy—can enjoy the same kind of weight-loss success as I've had. They say they can't spend eight hours exercising every day, like I did at the ranch on *The Biggest Loser*. You don't have to! The best lesson I learned from our trainer, Bob Harper, was to work within my capabilities. I couldn't run, so I walked. When my knees were hurting so badly that I couldn't walk,

he put me in the pool so I could swim. Or he sat me down and had me do arm exercises with light weights.

If you're used to sitting all day and doing nothing, then any activity—even if it's taking a short walk or taking a ballroom dancing class—will make a difference. The key is to get moving in any way that you can. Of course you should check with your doctor before you start any new routine. But it helps to think small. Take it one step at a time. That's what I did, and I walked a marathon.

EXCUSE: *Fat is hereditary in my family. Everybody's big.*
THE TRUTH: So what?! Everybody in my family was big. Now we're smaller. Genetics are not forcing you to eat a bag of junk from a drive-through. Your DNA is not telling you to sit on the couch and eat ice cream or chips.

True, some people are naturally thin, no matter what they eat. Good for them. All you can do is work with what you've got.

Becky and I talk about this frequently. We believe that genetics does make some people more prone to weight gain. But we can't use that as an excuse. This also comes up when parents say their chubby child is going to "grow" into his or her metabolism by having a growth spurt and suddenly slimming down.

That won't happen if the kid is eating fast food and sugary snacks all day long.

EXCUSE: *I have aches and pains. I can't even go out for a walk.*
THE TRUTH: Michael walked 26.2 miles despite excruciating hip pain. I had a torn rotator cuff when we went to the ranch. A professional trainer can show you safe ways to work around your disability, such as exercising in a swimming pool without stressing your joints.

EXCUSE: *I don't have time to exercise or cook healthy foods.*
THE TRUTH: If your doctor said you had cancer and you needed to spend an hour every night in chemotherapy to save your life, you'd find the time.

Eating healthy food and exercising is the best way to cure your ailments and prevent other ones from setting in and shortening your life. The time you invest now to eat healthily and exercise will pay off in the long run when you live a longer, healthier life.

Did you know that obese people die an average of twelve years earlier than normal-weight people? That's according to a study in the online journal *Obesity.*

The Biggest Loser was the fountain of youth for me. When I arrived at the ranch, I was the "sickest contestant," taking fourteen pills and 50 units of insulin a day. Just months later, I was down to one pill and no shots.

That's a magic cure if I ever heard of one!

Still not convinced? Talk to someone with diabetes or high blood pressure whose kidneys have failed as a result. Ask them how many hours and days a week they sit hooked up to a dialysis machine. Then compare that amount of time to the hours you would need to write a grocery list, shop, and prepare the vegetables and grilled or roasted lean meats.

Doctor visits. Surgeries. Diagnostic tests. Think about it: a healthy lifestyle actually saves you time in the long run.

EXCUSE: *Healthy food is too expensive. The dollar menu at fast-food places saves me so much money.*
THE TRUTH: How much do you spend on prescription medications every month? How often do you have to go out and buy bigger clothes? Is your furniture breaking because

you're so heavy? Were you like me and Becky, buying *three* airplane seats for *two* people?

Obviously, it's less expensive to buy healthy foods than to finance a fat lifestyle.

Any other thinking is penny-wise, pound-foolish. You can go to a local farmers' market and buy a ton of fresh fruits, vegetables, and herbs for super-low prices. Frozen vegetables are just as healthy and are often on sale in bulk at the grocery store. Better yet, grow a garden; it's practically free!

EXCUSE: *My kids won't eat vegetables or fruit.*
THE TRUTH: If the kids get hungry enough, and the only snacks around are apples, bananas, and grapes, I guarantee they'll eat them—and love them. Fruit is nature's candy. It's sweet, the colors are fun, and it's filling.

As for vegetables, you can make them fun or consult cookbooks that show delicious ways to serve them.

If Becky and I could turn back the clock and do it all over again, we would have insisted that the boys eat fruits and vegetables from the time they started on solid foods. They would have been used to the tastes and textures, and have continued eating these healthy foods after they were old enough to make their own choices.

The bottom line is that you're the parent. You do the shopping. And you have the power to serve healthy foods to your kids.

EXCUSE: *I eat when I'm stressed. Or bored. I can't break my bad habits.*
THE TRUTH: You can train your brain to do something else when you're stressed or bored. Or you can make

a healthier food choice if you must indulge your nervous munching. Your success is all about choices inspired by your overall goal of feeling better and looking better.

It's not easy, but it's worth it. To this day, every time I get in the car, I think, "Where can I stop and get something to eat?" Back when I was obese, I did that every day. A bag of burgers and fries here, a couple candy bars there. You name it—I ate it in my car.

Talk about a habit. For foodaholics, the car is the equivalent of a drug den for a drug addict. It's secret. It's sneaky. And it has bad consequences.

Now, when I get in the car, I answer that question with, "Nowhere. You already ate lunch," or "Eat that apple you brought from home."

It's not easy. Sometimes I have to take it minute by minute to stop myself from turning into the drive-through. I just keep driving, and I'm glad I did.

EXCUSE: *If I stray one bite off my diet, I lose control and binge.*
THE TRUTH: You can stop this cycle. Becky and I were both like this. But what I learned on the ranch was that if I screwed up once, so what? I'd have to get right back on my program. Now if I overindulge at lunchtime, I don't use it as a license to eat junk the rest of the day. And I no longer think I'm a rotten guy for blowing it. Instead I eat a sensible supper and do some gardening to stay active.

Here's an example. The other day, when Becky and I were playing euchre with friends, I ate more than I should have, including the snack mix on the tables. Becky made some chocolate bars, and I had a couple. I ate like everyone else there.

The next day, I stuck to my regimen and compensated for the

extra calories by walking more and eating less. I've convinced myself that this is what "thin America" thinks. It's a mind game. And I'm winning.

So what do I eat on a typical day?

For breakfast, it's usually four eggs with Parmesan cheese. On the weekends, I enjoy an omelet with Becky at one of our favorite restaurants. But now I bring the hash browns home and feed them to our dogs. Lunch and dinner? Ron's Famous Turkey Burgers.

I snack on apples, watermelon, and grapes between meals. In the evenings, we use the air popper for popcorn.

My weight is holding steady in the mid two hundreds. This is the closest relationship to normal I've ever had with food and weight. And I love it. Some days I'm on autopilot, and food just isn't an issue. Other days it's a real struggle.

I have to play mind games with myself to stay on track. I equate eating junk in mass quantities with early death.

Once you stop making excuses and let go of the fear, you can beat obesity too.

CHAPTER 16

/ **FIT FAMILY**

We're Beating Obesity,
and You Can Too

Some days it's a struggle.

And we mean *struggle*.

Minute by minute, we fight the urge to soothe stressed-out feelings with ice cream, pizza, or cheeseburgers. Sometimes we still feel fat in our minds, as if our brains haven't caught up with our new bodies. That is a horrible—and dangerous—mental place to be. Because when we were at our biggest, we felt trapped by hopelessness that we would never lose weight. In that mind-set, eating everything in sight was okay, because it didn't really matter.

But when your body is thin and your mind is still "fat," it takes tremendous resolve to not eat recklessly. Call it the food-aholic beast whispering to Ron to eat peanut butter, or telling Becky to eat chocolate, or Max to chow down on fast food, or Michael to scarf down cookies.

We may never slay our food addictions. But we have learned to control them.

Our determination to never go back to being an unhealthy and unhappy obese family is a powerful force against the beast. That determination pushes us through those moments of struggle and stops us from going back to our bad habits.

The demons are always there, but we're all committed to making this a permanent change in our lives.

One day at a time. Sometimes one *hour* at a time.

What works for us can work for anyone. Without a million-dollar gym. Without world-famous personal trainers. And without a prime-time TV show.

One thing that sums up our lifestyle change since the show happened when friends were hanging out at our house. One of the guys opened our refrigerator to grab a beer. In shock, he yelled: "Hey! What happened? There are vegetables in your beer drawer!"

We always laugh at this story because it shows how we have completely changed what we keep in the house and how we live. Vegetables in the beer drawer. If that's what it takes, then that's what we'll keep doing, because we're finally beating obesity. And if we can do it—then so can you!

Staples in Our Kitchen

Boneless, skinless chicken breast
Sliced, low-sodium chicken breast
Extra-lean ground turkey
White tuna
Egg Beaters
Frozen vegetables: broccoli, spinach, stir-fry blend
Frozen berries
Light whole wheat bread
High-fiber, low-calorie tortillas
Whole wheat sandwich buns
Brown rice
Low-fat cheese: Swiss, American, feta
Light yogurt
Salad blend lettuces: romaine, field greens
Low-calorie, low-sodium pasta sauce
Low-calorie salad dressing packets: raspberry vinaigrette,
    honey mustard
Popcorn (for air-popping)
Lemons

Seasoning: hot sauce, salt-free mixed seasonings (a variety)
Nonstick cooking spray

To put it simply, we eat very simply.

The following recipes are not meant to be culinary master-pieces; they are just some of the dishes that we eat regularly and that are healthy and quick. Some contain calorie counts and others don't.

Recipes

Egg Wrap

½ cup of egg substitute (such as Egg Beaters)
80-calorie high-fiber tortilla (we like La Tortilla Factory)
Salt-free seasoning of choice (I like Southwest)
1 slice low-fat cheese

Spray pan with nonstick cooking spray. Pour egg substitute in hot pan and cook until set. Top the tortilla with the cooked eggs, the seasoning, and slice of cheese. Fold in the edges of the tortilla and roll up.

This is packed with fiber and protein for less than 200 calories and is easy to make and eat on the go.

Vegetable Soup

1 large yellow onion, diced
¼ cabbage, chopped
2 zucchini squash, cut in bite-size pieces
8 oz. sliced mushrooms
Salt-free herb seasoning
1 tsp. minced garlic

8 cups low-sodium chicken or vegetable stock
1 can diced tomatoes
2 lbs. frozen vegetables of choice

In a large stockpot coated with nonstick cooking spray, sauté onion, cabbage, and zucchini until soft. Add mushrooms and continue to cook. Add seasoning and garlic. When vegetables are tender, add stock and tomatoes. Add frozen vegetables and simmer until frozen vegetables are cooked.

Once the soup is finished, I like to take 2 cups of the broth and vegetables and puree it; then add it back into the pot to make it thicker. If your kids don't like chunks of veggies, you can puree the entire recipe, making it very thick and smooth.

Turkey Meatloaf

1½ lbs. lean ground turkey
3 slices light, high-fiber whole wheat bread, processed into crumbs
⅓ cup chicken broth
1 medium onion, diced small
1 carrot, shredded
1 8 oz. package of mushrooms, finely chopped
2 cloves garlic, minced
½ cup egg substitute
1 tbsp. Worcestershire sauce

Topping:

½ cup tomato sauce
1 tbsp. mustard
1 tbsp. Worcestershire sauce
1 tbsp. brown sugar

Preheat oven to 350°F.

Mix the turkey and the remaining ingredients (except topping). Divide the mixture into two and form two loaves. Place on a foil-lined, rimmed baking sheet.

Mix the remaining topping ingredients and spread evenly over the two loaves.

Bake for 50–60 minutes (until internal temperature is 165°F).

Let rest for 10 minutes before slicing.

Turkey Tacos

1 1b. lean ground turkey
Salt-free Southwest seasoning
Low-calorie, high-fiber tortillas
Salsa
Shredded lettuce
Fat-free sour cream
Fat-free shredded cheese

Brown turkey and add seasoning to taste. Add favorite toppings to make tacos. Simple but nutritious!

Simple Grilled Chicken

I make grilled chicken at the beginning of the week for dinner, but I make way more than we'll need and use it throughout the week to take for lunch for a salad topper.

Flatten boneless, skinless chicken breasts.

Take about ½ tsp. of olive oil and rub it on clean hands; then rub chicken to lightly coat so it won't stick to pan or grill plate.

Season with salt-free seasoning of choice (lemon pepper, garlic herb, Southwest, citrus herb, etc.).

Heat up a countertop grill or pan. Cook through (about 6 minutes per side).

Lemon Aioli Dipping Sauce

1 lemon, juiced
½ cup of low-fat mayo
1 tsp. minced garlic
1 tbsp. of fresh herbs (I like finely chopped rosemary or basil)

Squeeze the lemon juice into the mayonnaise and stir in the garlic and herbs. Let sit to blend flavors.

Use as a dipping sauce for chicken or asparagus.

Roasted Asparagus Parmesan

Preheat oven to 375°F.

Take one bunch of asparagus and trim tough ends: Break one stalk where it naturally bends, then just take the rest of the bunch and cut off at the same point.

Toss with 1 tsp. of olive oil and sprinkle with salt-free seasoning.

Spread on parchment-lined pan and roast for 15 minutes.

Remove from oven and sprinkle with 2 tbsps. of shredded Parmesan cheese.

Sweet Potato Wedges

Preheat oven to 375°F.

Cut whole sweet potatoes in half lengthwise; then take each half and cut into long wedges.

Toss the wedges in 1 tbsp. of olive oil until lightly covered.

Sprinkle with salt-free seasoning and roast until tender (about 30–40 minutes).

Michigan Cherry Salad

Field greens
2 tbsps. dried cherries
¼ cup mandarin oranges
Red onion slivers
1 oz. fat-free feta cheese
3 oz. grilled chicken
1 50-calorie packet of fat-free raspberry vinaigrette

Combine ingredients in medium bowl. Add vinaigrette and toss to coat.

Quick Italian-Style Chicken

Make the Simple Grilled Chicken using an Italian-blend seasoning.

Top with warm low-calorie pasta sauce, 2 tbsps. fat-free mozzarella, and 1 tbsp. of Parmesan cheese. Cover skillet and warm until cheese melts.

Turkey Burgers

1 lb. extra-lean ground turkey

Season turkey with cayenne pepper, onion powder, and black pepper. (If sodium isn't an issue, experiment and mix with dry soup mix—makes lots of different flavors.)

Form into 4 oz. patties.

These freeze well.

Ron's Filet Mignon,
as Seen on *The Biggest Loser*

During the episode when the other team went to the spa, our four-member team prepared a feast in the kitchen at the ranch. Here's how.

The menu: filet mignon, roasted asparagus, salad, and sweet potatoes.

5 oz. cuts of filet mignon
Black pepper
Salad greens (with vinaigrette or other low-calorie dressing)
Raw asparagus
Sweet potatoes
Butter spray
Stevia sweetener
Cinnamon

Sprinkle filets with black pepper and cook on a grill to preferred wellness.

Place asparagus on a cookie sheet and cook in oven preheated to 400°F. Check after 12 minutes and keep checking until desired wellness is achieved. You can roast any type of vegetable—broccoli, peppers, cauliflower, zucchini, etc.—this way.

Wrap sweet potatoes in paper towels and microwave for six minutes. Cut in half; each person gets half a sweet potato. Spray with butter spray and sprinkle with stevia and cinnamon. They taste like candy!

Mike's Yogurt Sauces,
as Seen on *The Biggest Loser*

Mike became a master at creating sauces for a variety of tastes. All it takes is some plain, nonfat Greek-style yogurt and a bit of creativity to whip up what you like. For example:

Faux tartar sauce for fish:

Add a bit of lemon juice and pepper to Greek yogurt; it's the perfect sauce for fish.

Mexican spread/dip:

Mix Mrs. Dash chipotle seasoning with Greek yogurt. Spread over a corn tortilla or use as a dip for cubed, baked chicken breasts.